D1236688

Against Bioethics

Basic Bioethics

Glenn McGee and Arthur Caplan, editors

Against Bioethics

Jonathan Baron

The MIT Press
Cambridge, Massachusetts
London, England

MIT Press books may be purchased at special quantity discounts for business or sales promotional use. For information, please e-mail special_sales@ mitpress.mit.edu or write to Special Sales Department, The MIT Press, 55 Hayward Street, Cambridge, MA 02142–1315.

This book was set in Palatino by the author.
Printed on recycled paper.
Printed and bound in the United States of America.

Library of Congress Cataloging-in-Publication Data

Baron, Jonathan
Against bioethics / Jonathan Baron
    p. cm. — (Basic bioethics series)
Includes bibliographical references and index.
ISBN 0–262–02596–5 (hc. : alk. paper)
1. Medical ethics—philosophy. 2. Medical ethics—Decision making.
3. Decision making. 4. Informed consent (Law) 5. Duress (Law)
I. Title. II. Series.

R725.5B25 2006
174.2—dc22

2005054484

10   9   8   7   6   5   4   3   2   1

Contents

Series Foreword

We are pleased to present the nineteenth book in the series Basic Bioethics. The series presents innovative works in bioethics to a broad audience and introduces seminal scholarly manuscripts, state-of-the-art reference works, and textbooks. Such broad areas as the philosophy of medicine, advancing genetics and biotechnology, end-of-life care, health and social policy, and the empirical study of biomedical life are engaged.

Glenn McGee
Arthur Caplan

Basic Bioethics Series Editorial Board
Tod S. Chambers
Susan Dorr Goold
Mark Kuczewski
Herman Saatkamp

Preface

This book brings together three of my long-standing interests: decision analysis, utilitarianism, and applied bioethics. I have felt for some time that decision analysis needed firm roots in utility theory and in the sophisticated forms of utilitarian philosophy advocated by Richard Hare and others. I have watched the recent growth of applied bioethics, at first through the eyes of two close colleagues, David Asch and Peter Ubel, and as a member of the Ethics Committee of the Hospital of the University of Pennsylvania and the Institutional Review Board. I became more and more disturbed about how bioethicists were neglecting medical decision analysis. With my increased involvement with the journal *Medical Decision Making*, I saw how decision analysis was developing, and it seems highly relevant to questions faced in bioethics. I think decision analysis should get more attention from both the medical and policy-making communities.

So this book arose as an expression of my grumpiness about what is happening and not happening—in these worlds. I have retained the grumpy title and a few rants (mostly against Institutional Review Boards, which may yet drive me out of empirical research before I am ready to retire from it). But basically I try to present an explication, in very rough outline, of what applied bioethics might look like if it took utilitarian decision analysis more seriously.

I also include some psychology here. That is my field, and I do explain at least why I think that many moral intuitions are interesting psychological phenomena rather than windows into some sort of moral truth.

Many of the ideas here have benefited from discussions with David Asch, David Casarett, Andy (Andrea) Gurmankin, Jason Karlawish, Josh Metlay, Peter Ubel, and other members of David Asch's lab meeting. I thank Laura Damschroder, Neal Dawson, Daniel Wikler, and especially Andy Gurmankin and three anonymous reviewers for comments on a draft.

Chapter 1

Introduction

On September 17, 1999, Jesse Gelsinger died at the age of 18 as a result of participating in a medical experiment at the Hospital of the University of Pennsylvania. Gelsinger had a mild form of a rare metabolic disorder called ornithine transcarbamylase deficiency (a missing enzyme), a condition he could control with drugs and a low-protein diet. The severe form of the disease caused infants to die a few weeks after birth. Dr. James Wilson of the University of Pennsylvania had a promising therapy for the disorder and wanted to try it. The therapy involved replacing defective genes with genes that would produce the enzyme. The replacement involved injecting a virus (adenovirus) that had the relevant gene. The therapy was promising not only because it might cure this disease but also because it was one of the first tests of gene therapy itself, a general method that could treat a variety of diseases. It was risky, though, because the virus itself could cause trouble.

For reasons that are still unclear, the therapy went awry, and Gelsinger died from multiple organ failure. In hindsight, it became clear that many errors were made. Gelsinger was not fully informed of the risks. Wilson had apparently failed to report less serious problems with other patients that might have led officials to look more carefully at the proposed experiment. Plus, Wilson had a financial interest in its success. (The relevance and seriousness of these errors, and others, has been disputed: see Miller 2000.) As a result of these errors, Wilson's entire institute was prevented from doing research on human subjects, and rules were tightened all over the United States (and possibly in other countries too). The investigation of this case is still going on, six years later.

Note, though, that Gelsinger was reasonably healthy and did not need the therapy. He agreed to be a subject because he wanted to help the infants. (He said to a friend, "What's the worst that could happen to me? I die, and it's for the babies" [Stolberg 1999].) But the babies would die anyway. Why couldn't the new therapy be tested on them? It could do no harm, and it might work.

There were reasons for using an adult (personal communication from Arthur Caplan, Aug. 23, 2002). First, the logistics of using babies would be difficult. The experiment would have to be done quickly after suitable subjects were identified. Evidently, though, the logistical problems were not so great as to prevent the researchers from initially thinking about an experiment on babies.

Second, the trial was a "phase 1" trial, which means that its "purpose" was to assess side effects, dosage, and so on. And it would be difficult to assess side effects in babies, who would live for a shorter amount of time than adults, if the therapy failed to help. The rules did not allow anyone to consider the possibility (however remote) that the therapy might actually have helped. Because there was officially no benefit (because the official purpose was not to assess benefit, although benefit could have easily been assessed), fully informed consent was required according to United States regulations (e.g., Department of Health and Human Services 2002).

Given this second constraint, the question was whether parents could consent. It was concluded that they could not. Why? Because they were "coerced" by their child's disease into agreeing (Miller 2000). Or perhaps because they were under such stress that they could not decide rationally in the very short time that they would have.

Notice that I use the passive, "it was concluded." The responsibility for this principle is difficult to locate. Wilson's team had initially proposed to try the experiment on infants. Miller (2000) blames the Food and Drug Administration, but Wilson had apparently engaged in self-censorship and did not even get as far as asking the FDA. Rather, he was advised by the director of Penn's Bioethics Center, Arthur Caplan, that using infants would not fly. Caplan has said that he was not giving his own opinion about what should be done but simply informing Wilson of the consensus view in the field of bioethics.

I do not want to dwell further on the facts of this case. That would take at least another book. Rather, I want to discuss the principles involved. Suppose it is true that the experiment could have been tried on infants who would have died anyway.

In what sense are parents "coerced" into agreeing? The relevant sense is that the therapy has a very low but nonzero probability of a large benefit—that is, saving their infants—and a low probability of causing a small harm, such as allowing the parents to keep false hopes alive for a few more days or weeks. Faced with such a decision, many rational people would consent. The prohibition of the research on infants took that decision from them; someone knew better what was in their best interest.

Such an offer of benefit shares one feature with true coercion. If I point a gun at you and say, "Your money or your life," it is reasonable for you to give me your money. Any rational person would do it, just as any rational person would accept the offer of a potentially life-saving therapy. So coercion involves presenting people with decisions that a rational person would make only one way, but the converse does not follow: decisions that can be rationally made one way are not necessarily all coercive.

What is the difference? Coercion seems to involve a threat of a loss. But that is not quite right, because "loss" and "gain" are relative terms. I shall argue later that the critical difference is that coercion involves the threat of a net loss for everyone relative to the status quo, what economists call a "deadweight loss." True coercion is sometimes necessary, as when we threaten punishment to prevent crime; but it is not a good way to recruit subjects for medical experiments.

In sum, it is conceivable that the death of Jesse Gelsinger was the result of an error in reasoning, a confusion on the part of almost everyone involved. It may have resulted from a principle of bioethics.

Such errors are found throughout the enterprise of applied bioethics. Of course, bioethicists who influence these outcomes would not admit to errors. I shall argue here, though, that they truly are making errors.

1.1   What this book tries to do

The principles of coercion and informed consent are examples of a set of principles applied by the new field of applied bioethics. These principles sometimes have the force of law, yet some of these were not adopted by any legislature nor promulgated by any regulatory agency. They come from a kind of consensus among people who call themselves bioethicists. Bioethicists have some form of academic training, usually in philosophy. However, the field of applied bioethics has to some extent taken on a life of its own, with its own degree programs, local consultants, and committees. It is this applied field that I am "against." It has become a kind of secular priesthood to which governments and other institutions look for guidance, but it lacks the authority that comes from a single, coherent guiding theory in which practitioners are trained.

It is interesting to contrast bioethics and economics. Today, economists advise governments, corporations, and universities, and they are taken seriously (although one might argue not seriously enough). Economics has a coherent theory of what it is doing, and the theory has withstood empirical challenge, or modified its assumptions in response to evidence. Economists cannot predict the future all that well, but they can give the best advice there is about how to make decisions under uncertainty, and they can explain at length why it is, in fact, the best advice.

Applied bioethics, by contrast, tends either to be suspicious of theory, or else it attempts to apply different, sometimes competing, theories (Caplan 1992; Wikler 1994). The major text in the field, Beauchamp and Childress (1983, and subsequent editions), presents utilitarian and deontological (non-utilitarian) theories as if they were both relevant, despite their divergent positions on many issues. In practice, bioethical advice tends to be based on tradition and intuitive judgments. Often, its advice is reasonable and leads to good outcomes. But, as in the Gelsinger case, we might well ask where these judgments get their authority to override considerations of consequences. If the consequences of a decision are clearly expected to be worse—as in the case of testing the therapy on healthy adults instead of babies who had nothing to lose—where do bioethicists get the authority to cause harm?

It could have a coherent theory paired with an expertise in the knowledge of that theory. Namely, it could embrace utilitarianism. Utilitarianism holds that the best option is the one that does the most expected good ("maximizes expected utility"). Such a theory would never yield decisions that clearly go against the good of those involved, such as the decision to use healthy adults in the experiment. Expertise is involved in less clear cases because the prediction of expected good is often complex and far from obvious. Utilitarianism, when applied, draws on economic theory, which also makes predictions of expected good in complex situations.

It also draws on an applied field called decision analysis, which, in turn, is based on decision theory, a mathematical approach to the analysis of decisions. Indeed, the discipline of decision analysis is the closest thing to applied utilitarianism. Decision theory, like utilitarianism, defines the best option as the one that does the most expected good. The main difference between what is called utilitarianism and what is called decision theory is that the latter does not usually concern itself with trade-offs across people, where one option is good for one person and another option for another person. But the theory can be extended to handle this case.

I should note that decision analysis, as practiced, often takes nonutilitarian factors into account, that is, factors, such as fairness, that do not concern the good of any individual people. But I shall stick mainly to the limited form of decision analysis that considers only the good of individuals, with no separate idea of "social good" except for the sum of what is good for individuals.

I should also note that much of the scholarship in bioethics is, in fact, based on utilitarian theory and looks favorably on that theory. I am, as I have said, talking about bioethics as it is applied, not scholarship. Perhaps the utilitarian scholarly writings would have more influence on practice if they were combined with the tools of decision analysis.

In this book, I want to discuss several issues that engage bioethics today, and then show how these issues can be illuminated by applied utilitarianism, in the form of decision analysis. Thus, what I have to say is "against bioethics" but it is also "for" an alternative.

I shall not carry out a formal decision analysis of every issue. Indeed, I shall sketch such analyses for only a few issues. This is not a textbook of decision analysis.[1] Rather, I shall point to the relevant elements of decisions that would have to be included in an analysis. In some cases, it is clear that some of these elements are very difficult to quantify, and a full decision analysis requires quantification. For example, a decision may hinge on some value that is difficult to measure, such as the harm that is done to a person when his wishes are violated after his death. In such cases, I think it is still a contribution to point out where the difficulty is. The fact that we have trouble measuring this value does not imply that it doesn't exist, and it does not imply that it no longer determines the answer about what we should do. If we make the decision in some way other than by using our best guess about the quantity in question, then the decision-analytic approach tells us the conditions under which we would make the wrong choice.

It is surely true that the subjective estimation of values and probabilities required for decision analysis is prone to error. The question is, compared to what? (This is a common question asked in decision theory.) The alternative is often some rule. Yet, in many cases, the rule is almost certain to make even greater errors. For example, as I shall discuss later, the decision about fetal testing should, according to decision analysis, depend heavily on the mother's values concerning birth defects, miscarriage, and abortion (Kupperman et al. 1999). Surely, better decisions would result from even a crude attempt to measure such values—even so crude as asking the mother how she feels about these outcomes—rather than from imposing some fixed rule on everyone, such as "amniocentesis after age 35." In other cases, the alternative is not a fixed rule but someone's intuitive judgment. We have learned that such judgments are both highly variable from person to person and also subject to systematic biases (Baron 2000).

Decision analysis is also difficult and time consuming. I shall not be recommending, though, that it be done very often. Rather, I shall argue that our thinking about issues should be informed by its perspective. This is why, in this book, I shall dwell mostly on discussions of what is relevant in decision analysis and what is not.

---

[1] For that, see: Baron 2000 for a quick introduction. Some of the many introductions are: Keeney and Raiffa 1993; von Winterfeldt and Edwards 1986; and Hunink et al. 2001.

I shall also make use of the general perspective on decision making that utilitarian decision analysis provides. This perspective is quantitative: it makes distinctions between large and small benefits, between large and small harms, and between high and low probabilities, even in the absence of precise quantification. It is thus less likely to suffer from being penny wise and pound foolish. It also looks at the big picture, focusing on all consequences; it can do this because it thinks of good and harm quantitatively so that they can be compared across different kinds of outcomes. It does not isolate immediate effects, or effects that are psychologically salient. It also compares possible options to each other, not to some nonexistent utopian ideal, nor just to the status quo or the result of doing nothing. Finally, it is future oriented; decisions, after all, affect the future, not the past. This general perspective provides us with a useful way to think about decisions, even if we do not make use of a single number.

Similar to economic theory, decision analysis need not have the last word. Economists don't usually control policy. They do provide the background assumptions for policymakers. If bioethics were to take decision analysis as its basis, it would have the authority of a single, well-reasoned theory, an authority it now lacks. If officials then wanted to override its recommendations, they would at least know what they were doing. Decision analysis will not provide a philosophy on which everyone could agree, but the usefulness of a theory may have little to do with its consensual acceptability (Wikler 1994). People do not agree about economic theory either.

If, on the other hand, decision analysis came to be trusted as a theory, consequences for people would be better, because producing the best consequences is the goal of decision analysis. Perhaps there is some reason against this, in morality or religion, but good consequences are, by definition, good. So giving them up for the sake of some other principle at least requires a difficult trade. Trust in decision analysis, like trust in modern medicine, economics, or other sciences, takes time to develop.

In the next chapter, I shall sketch very briefly a point of view on some of the history and principles of bioethics. Then, I shall describe the basic argument for utilitarianism and its use in decision analysis. I shall not do this in detail. Subsequent chapters will raise some of the subtle issues, and a full explication of these theories is well beyond the limited scope of this book. But I shall at least try to show that the theory does have a foundation.

The rest of the book will examine illustrative issues chosen mostly because they are of current interest to me and many others. In the conclusion, I try to take a somewhat broader view of the implications of utilitarianism for health and human well-being in general.

Chapter 2

Bioethics vs. Utilitarianism

Bioethics is a recent phenomenon. It is an attempt to develop institutions that help people make difficult decisions about health care, health research, and other research and applications in biology, such as genetic engineering of crops. It draws on moral philosophy, law, and some of its own traditions. These traditions take the form of documents and principles that grew out of the Nuremberg trials after World War II. In some cases, these documents have acquired the force of law, but in most cases the principles are extralegal—that is, enforced by general agreement. Bioethics now has its own journals and degree programs. You can make a living (with difficulty) as a bioethicist.

As a field, bioethics plays three roles somewhat analogous to medicine. It is an applied discipline. People trained in bioethics work in hospitals and other medical settings, sometimes for pay, to help staff and patients think about difficult decisions. I was, for several years, a member of the Ethics Committee of the Hospital of the University of Pennsylvania. This committee had no full-time paid staff but it did draw on various administrative resources of the hospital. We had monthly meetings that consisted of case presentations—usually reports of cases that were settled—and sometimes more general presentations. Members of the committee were on call for quickly arranged "consults," in which four or five members would meet with medical staff and patient representatives (and rarely the patient herself) over some difficult decision. The most common involved "pulling the plug," but other decisions involved matters such as whether to turn a patient out of the hospital, given that she was no longer in need of hospital services but still unable to live on her own because of a combination of incompetence, poverty, and lack of others who might help her. Some members of this committee had taken courses in bioethics, but most had no special training. Nonetheless, the committee saw its work as informed by the tradition of applied bioethics as I discuss it here.

The second role is academic. As I noted, bioethics has its own journals and societies, and some universities have departments of bioethics, or parts of departments devoted to it. I have almost nothing to say about the academic side of bioethics. The literature is huge, and it would take me too far afield. Some contributors to this literature would agree with things that I say here; others would dispute them. Many are utilitarians (although few of these are involved with decision analysis). There is no consensus. The consensus arises when the bioethics literature is distilled into its final common path—that is, the actual influence of bioethical discussion on outcomes, and that will be my focus.

The third role is in the formulation of codes of ethics. Here the situation is somewhat unique, since most codes of ethics are written by the practitioners to whom the codes apply. When it comes to the ethics of research, in particular, a certain tension arises between researchers and those nonresearchers who write the rules. The tension plays out largely in the review boards that examine research proposals (chapter 7).

2.1   History: Nuremberg and Tuskegee

The history of bioethics follows a pattern that may explain many human rules, both social and personal. Some catastrophe happens, then people look for some rule that would have prevented the catastrophe if the rule had been in effect. Then they implement the rule. The problem is that they do not think much about whether the rule may also prevent other things that would not be so bad in its absence, or whether the rule will prevent the next catastrophe.

Modern bioethics began largely with the discovery of Nazi abuses committed in the name of medical research prior to and during World War II. Prisoners in concentration camps—who were imprisoned largely because of their ethnic background or their political views—were subjected to horrendous and harmful procedures. They had no choice, but of course their options had already been sharply limited by their imprisonment. (Similar studies went on with conscientious objectors in the United States—such as the starvation studies of Keys and Keys—but most of these subjects had more options.)

These abuses were uncovered at the Nuremberg war-crimes trials after Germany's defeat (1945–1946). The court, as part of its verdict against several physicians involved in the experiments, proposed a set of principles (Trials of War Criminals ... 1949), which never acquired the force of law, but which has been the basis of all subsequent codes. The first principle of the "Nuremberg Code" was:

> The voluntary consent of the human subject is absolutely essential. This means that the person involved should have legal capacity to give consent; should be so situated as to be able to exercise free power of choice, without the intervention of any element of force, fraud, deceit, duress, overreaching, or other ulterior form of constraint or coercion; and should have sufficient knowledge and comprehension of the elements of the subject matter involved as to enable him to make an understanding and enlightened decision. This latter element requires that before the acceptance of an affirmative decision by the experimental subject there should be made known to him the nature, duration, and purpose of the experiment; the method and means by which it is to be conducted; all inconveniences and hazards reasonable to be expected; and the effects upon his health or person which may possibly come from his participation in the experiment.

Although this principle sounds reasonable, its subsequent interpretation has led to rules that have made things worse, such as the rules that prevented infants from being subjects in the experiment that killed Jesse Gelsinger, and a three-year moratorium on much emergency research in the United States (section 6.4).

The Nuremberg Code inspired later codes, in particular the Declaration of Helsinki of 1964 (World Medical Organization 1996) and the Belmont Report (National Commission for the Protection of Human Sub-

jects 1979). The last of these was in part a response to the Tuskegee
study of syphilis, in which 600 black men, 400 of whom had syphilis,
were monitored from 1932 to 1972, without treatment, to observe the
natural course of this lifelong, debilitating disease, even though an effective treatment (penicillin) became available in the 1950s. The experiment
ended as a result of press coverage. In 1974, partly as a result of this
coverage, the United States Congress passed the National Research Act,
which, among other things, appointed a commission to produce a report.
The resulting Belmont Report has been the basis of United States policy,
although, like the Nuremberg Code, it never acquired the force of law
(National Commission for the Protection of Human Subjects 1979). The
1974 act also mandated Institutional Review Boards (IRBs) for reviewing human subjects research in institutions that received United States
government funds.[1]

Many national governments, and the United Nations, have established formal bodies to deal with bioethical questions. Some were created because of some immediate concern but then went on to address
other issues. For example, in the United States, President George W.
Bush created the President's Council on Bioethics largely to help him
decide what to do about stem cell research, but the Council has now
produced several reports dealing with other issues, such as the use of
biotechnology to increase happiness. The United Nations Educational,
Scientific and Cultural Organization (UNESCO) has a bioethics section
that coordinates the activities of member states, most of which have their
own bioethics advisory committees or agencies. In the United States, individual states have bioethics panels. Universities run degree programs
in bioethics, and their graduates are employed in hospitals, government
agencies, and professional societies.

2.2 Principles of bioethics

Most introductions to bioethics provide an overview of various philosophical approaches to morality but then conclude with some sort of list
of basic principles. Typical are those listed in the Belmont Report (Na-

---

[1]Fairchild and Bayer (1999) discuss critically the extensive use of Tuskegee as a source
of analogies in bioethics.

tional Commission for the Protection of Human Subjects 1979): respect for persons, beneficence (or nonmaleficence), and justice.[2] Other lists of principles are often provided, but these three seem to capture a great deal of what might be called the standard approach, even though the Belmont Report applies them only to questions about research.

Most of these principles arose in moral philosophy. For example, the idea of respect for persons was emphasized by Kant, beneficence by the utilitarians, and justice by Aristotle (and many others). But they were incorporated into bioethics often in response to specific violations, as in the case of the Nazi crimes. The response is of the form, "Can we find a principle that this particular crime or abuse violates?" Thus, most of the abuses violated respect for persons because the subjects did not freely consent (in the case of the Nazis) or were not informed (as in the Tuskegee study); they also violated nonmaleficence because harm was done.

The principles in question are surely good ideas when other considerations are equal. In real cases, they conflict with each other and sometimes even with themselves. I present them to illustrate how this might happen. Decision analysis is designed to resolve such conflicts by quantifying the relevant considerations: outcomes and their probabilities.

2.2.1 Respect for persons

"Respect for persons incorporates at least two ethical convictions: first, that individuals should be treated as autonomous agents, and second, that persons with diminished autonomy are entitled to protection. The principle of respect for persons thus divides into two separate moral requirements: the requirement to acknowledge autonomy and the requirement to protect those with diminished autonomy." We might call these principles autonomy and paternalism, respectively. The principle of autonomy implies that people should be able to make choices for themselves, after being fully informed.

---

[2]The quotations that follow are from the Belmont Report, Part B, "Basic ethical principles."

Clearly, these two principles conflict. People should free to decide, but the freedom can be overridden if their capacity is diminished. But they cannot be coerced either. Thus, the working out of these principles requires various subsidiary principles for deciding who is diminished and who is free from coercion. For example, children below a certain age or demented adults are assumed to have diminished capacity. Prisoners are sometimes considered to be in a coercive situation because they do not have the freedom to voluntarily consent to a research study, therefore they must not be given the choice of whether to consent.

Further efforts are required to define capacity when it isn't clear whether people have it. Does psychological depression count as diminished capacity? What about mild schizophrenia (or severe schizophrenia, for that matter)?

2.2.2 Beneficence

"Persons are treated in an ethical manner not only by respecting their decisions and protecting them from harm, but also by making efforts to secure their well-being. ... Two general rules have been formulated as complementary expressions of beneficent actions in this sense: (1) do not harm and (2) maximize possible benefits and minimize possible harms" (Belmont Report, Part B, National Commission for the Protection of Human Subjects 1979).

The "do no harm" maxim, originally from the Hippocratic oath, is often interpreted as meaning that "one should not injure one person regardless of the benefits that might come to others," but the Belmont Report argues that it is acceptable to increase the *risk* of harm to someone in order to help someone else (e.g., in research). Even the law considers an increase in the risk of harm as a harm in itself. The report seems to be attempting to balance risk of harm and risk of benefit, but it does this in a crude way.

The principle of beneficence also creates conflict: "A difficult ethical problem remains, for example, about research that presents more than minimal risk without immediate prospect of direct benefit to the children involved. Some have argued that such research is inadmissible, while others have pointed out that this limit would rule out much research promising great benefit to children in the future."

2.2.3 Justice

"An injustice occurs when some benefit to which a person is entitled is denied without good reason or when some burden is imposed unduly. Another way of conceiving the principle of justice is that equals ought to be treated equally." As the Belmont Report (Part B, National Commission for the Protection of Human Subjects 1979) notes, this statement begs the questions of what benefits or burdens are "due" or of what the measure of equality is (contribution, need, effort, merit, and so forth).

In practice, considerations of justice come up when, for example, research is done on poor subjects, who bear the risk, while the benefits of the research often accrue to rich patients who can pay for the resulting new technology. Thus, justice in practice is often a way of limiting further harm to those who are already down and out.

These three principles generate their own internal conflicts, but they also conflict with each other. Justice may demand punishment, but beneficence may demand mercy in the same case.

2.3 Bioethical principles vs. utilitarianism

The situation in applied bioethics is much like that in the law. We have superordinate principles either in the common law or a constitution. These principles are then made more specific by legislatures and courts, and more specific still by case law. Applied bioethics does not seem to have an analogue of case law.

More broadly, the same sort of cognitive processes are involved in the development of religious rules. Some case arises, judgments are made by applying known principles. These are weighed against each other somehow. Ultimately a new precedent is set. If a similar case uses the precedent, then a new, subordinate principle emerges (Hare 1952, ch. 4).

Much of the academic literature concerns the reconciliation of principles, but I shall deal with practice. In practice—for example, when review boards decide cases or when government agencies write regulations—the process is more intuitive. When principles conflict, people differ in their belief about which principle dominates. People may be especially attached to one principle or another, or chance factors may bring one property of a case or another to the front of each judge's mind. People may even consider consequences in the case at hand, weighing one consequence against another. The principle they then formulate— namely, "When we have this dilemma, horn A takes precedence over horn B"—may create worse consequences when the same dilemma arises in a different case.

In some cases, people consider more than one example before they attempt to state a general rule. For example, when stating the do-no-harm rule, the authors of the Belmont Report clearly considered the possibility that it might be good to harm some a little in order to help others a lot. They attempted to draw the line by saying that this was acceptable if the harm was uncertain. (The benefit of research is typically uncertain.)

Yet, uncertain harm to each of many research subjects amounts to almost certain harm to at least one subject. Does it matter that the identity of this person is unknown? Is it more acceptable to shoot someone if the shooter does not know the victim's name? Psychologically, the identified-victim effect is salient (Jenni and Loewenstein 1997), but this is easily understood in terms of the way we process information, which need not correspond either to moral rightness or best consequences (even assuming they aren't the same).

Principles of this sort do have one thing going for them, just as the law itself does: it is better to have some method for resolving disputes than none, and it is better if people can predict what judgments will be made about their behavior than if they cannot. Clear, public, principles are a lot better than nothing, even if the principles themselves are arbitrary.

A utilitarian approach can do what the law does—that is, provide a largely (but not perfectly) predictable way of settling difficult cases. It also is likely to produce better consequences. To put it simply, suppose that a utilitarian analysis says one thing and the application of bioethical principles, in the way usually done, says another. For example, suppose the issue is whether unconscious patients coming into an emergency room could be subjects for testing a life-saving procedure, given that they cannot consent. A utilitarian analysis—taking into account the probability that the procedure is effective, the (low but nonzero) probability that a person would not consent to it if given the chance, and the degree of resulting harm or benefit (utility) from the use of the procedure and the violation of the subject's wishes—says that the procedure should be tested, but an application of the rules (let us suppose) says it cannot be tested. The utilitarian analysis is by definition consistent with what each person would want, without knowing who he would be, but taking into account the probability that he would benefit from the treatment and the probability that he would object to the study. Thus, behind this sort of veil of ignorance, the utilitarian conclusion yields the best for everyone.

Thus, a situation could arise in which the overriding of a utilitarian conclusion makes everyone worse off. This is a simplistic example, but it illustrates a more general problem (Kaplow and Shavell 2002). The problem is, when we are in a situation like this, why should we make everyone worse off?

In more typical situations, we are viewing the situation *ex post*, after we know who is whom, so we are trading off the benefits/harms to some against the benefits/harms to others. How can we justify preventing a large harm to some people, for example, just because doing so will avoid a smaller harm to others? What can you tell the ones who would lose out? At least, in the utilitarian outcome, you can say, "I understand that you will lose here, but someone else will lose more if you don't." That is at least something to say. This is not a decisive argument for utilitarianism, of course. But it does point out the natural question that arises when any rule or principle goes against the utilitarian conclusion.

The second principle of beneficence, that we should maximize benefits and minimize harms, comes close to utilitarianism itself. The difference is that utilitarianism holds that "benefit" and "harm" are relative terms, which can be understood as upward or downward changes, respectively, on the same continuum of good (i.e., goodness or utility). Thus, harms and benefits can be compared with each other just as easily as benefits can be compared with benefits and harms with harms.

The first principle, "do no harm," is more difficult to justify, except for two things. First, most applications of this principle allow us to weasel out of the implication that harms of action are never justified by avoiding much greater harms of omission. The Belmont Report, for example, accepts the idea that the risk of harm is acceptable, even though a risk becomes a certainty.

Second, the modified principle (in which risks are allowed) might be a reasonable guide to action even though there are many cases in which it leads to the worse outcome. It could be seen as a kind of warning against overconfidence, such as might be exhibited by surgeons who deceive their patients into undergoing an experimental procedure that they deceive themselves into thinking will save many lives. Hare (1981) argues that such "intuitive" principles are often a good guide to action in everyday cases. Thus, to be a good utilitarian is sometimes to go against our own judgment of what would produce the best outcome, because we know that we must correct that judgment for systematic biases such as overconfidence.

I tend to think that this sort of argument—made extensively by Sidgwick (1962)—is too often used by utilitarian writers to justify their own conservative intuitions. Yet, whether this conservative argument is correct or not in a given case, my point here is that it serves as a utilitarian justification of the "do no harm" part of the principle of beneficence. And my general argument here is that all of the basic principles used in applied bioethics can be understood as having utilitarian roots.

Consider now the competing principles of autonomy and paternalism, both part of "respect for persons." Utilitarianism not only tells us why each of these is a good idea when other things are equal, but it also tells us how to think about the conflict between them. Autonomy is good because it allows people who are well informed and rational to make choices that maximize their own utility. In particular, each person tends to know her own values—her own utility function—better than others know it.

But some paternalism, at least in the form of expert advice, is justified when the person cannot get the relevant information about the relation between decision options and the utility of outcomes. Experts can also help by setting default options that are best for most people (Camerer et al. 2003; Sunstein and Thaler 2003). More extreme paternalism is warranted when the person will not follow good expert advice and when the effect of such advice is great. The utilitarian criterion here is whether we can expect the person (and anyone else affected) to be better off making her own judgment or having it made for her.

One other consideration is education. We sometimes allow people to make their own decisions even when we think they will not choose optimally because we want them to learn from experience. We must balance their future utility against their present disutility. This requires judgment, and that fact means that utilitarianism does not dictate the answer mechanically. But at least it tells us what judgment we ought to try to make.

Finally, consider justice. Its concern for the worse-off is rooted in utilitarianism combined with the declining marginal utility of goods. Most goods have less utility, the more of them we have. In the case of money the reason for this is simple. As we gain in a certain period of time, we rationally spend the money first on the things that are most important. Food before fashion. Thus, the first $100 gives us more utility than the last $100. Other goods show the same decline because of satiation. The first apple eaten is better than the fifth. There are exceptions to this rule; some goods—such as peanuts, perhaps—create increased desire for the same goods up to a point. But these are interesting only because they are rare, and they do not affect the general conclusion about the declining utility of money.

The principle of declining marginal utility by itself would prescribe equality in the allocation of money and other goods. If we start from equality and increase the wealth of one person at the expense of another, the gainer would gain less than the loser loses, in terms of what the money can buy. On the other side, if all money were distributed equally, then money could no longer provide an incentive to work. The amount of productive work would be reduced. Thus, the other side of justice is roughly the idea of equity as distinct from equality, that is, the idea (as stated by Aristotle in the *Nichomachean Ethics* and by many others since) that reward should be in proportion to contribution. The precise formula of proportionality is not necessarily the optimal incentive, but it is surely a reasonable approximation. Ideally, to maximize utility across all people, some sort of compromise between these two principles is needed, as is discussed at length in the theory of optimal taxation. For example, one common proposal is to tax income at a fixed percentage after subtracting some minimum amount.

Although the idea of equality and the idea of equity are both rooted in utilitarian theory, people may apply these ideas even when the utilitarian justification is absent. Greene and Baron (2001), for example, found that people want to distribute utility itself in the same way they would distribute money. They preferred distributions that were more equal. The subjects' judgments were internally inconsistent, because the subjects themselves judged that the utility of money was marginally declining, hence they should have taken this decline into account, if only a little, in their judgments of distributions of utility.

On the other side, Baron and Ritov (1993) found that people wanted to penalize companies for causing harm even when the size of the penalty would not affect compensation to the victim and when the penalty would provide no incentive for anyone to change behavior (because the penalty would be secret and the company that did the harm is going out of business anyway). The idea of penalties for causing harm is an application of the equity principle to the cases of losses. Possibly the same sort of result would be found for gains.

In sum, the basic principles of traditional ethics look a lot like heuristics designed to be rough guides to utility maximization—in other words, rules of thumb. When their utilitarian justification is not understood, they take on a life of their own, so that they are applied even in cases when the fail to maximize utility.

2.4   Rules and flowcharts

Many of the applications of bioethics result in rules that people are supposed to follow. The rules may concern when it is appropriate to waive informed consent to research, when to use a placebo control, when to accede to a patient's wish to die or forgo treatment, and so on. The rules are typically stated in a format that is supposed to be easy to implement— that is, a series of questions, each question yielding one of a small set of answers so that they may be put into a flowchart. Figure 2.1 shows a good example, one section of the rules that the University of Pennsylvania uses to decide whether a research proposal is exempt from formal review. (The term *exempt* is something of a euphemism, since a member of the IRB must review and approve the request to be exempt from review.)

This is a good example because the decisions at each step are fairly clear. (But what exactly is an educational survey? an observation of public behavior?) The use of rules in this form becomes more difficult when some of the categories require judgment about where the case falls on some continuum. The law is full of such examples, such as the standards

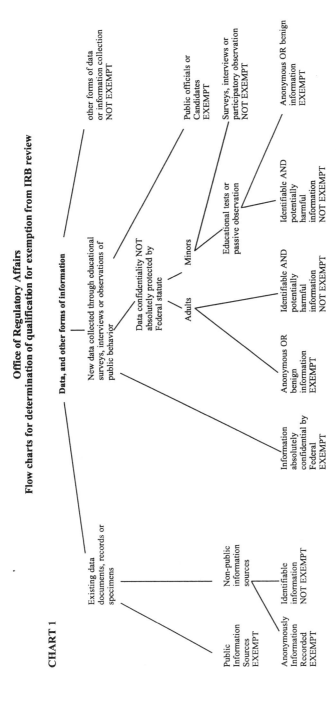

Figure 2.1: Partial flowchart for exemption from IRB review.

relevant to various kinds of legal cases: beyond a reasonable doubt, clear and convincing evidence, preponderance of the evidence, arbitrary and capricious, and so on. In the case of "beyond a reasonable doubt," for example, more certainty is surely better than less, but how much is required to meet that criterion? The criterion is vague. In the rules that result from bioethics, criteria are often stated in terms of risk and benefit, for example: high risk, minimal risk, substantial chance to benefit, and so on. The definition of minimal risk used at the University of Pennsylvania is "the probability and magnitude of harm or discomfort anticipated in the research are not greater than [sic] in and of themselves than those ordinarily encountered in daily life or during the performance of routine physical and psychological examinations or tests." The problem with this definition is that what is "routine" for one person is high risk for another. Do we consider this? If so, minimal risk for someone who lives in a high-crime neighborhood is much higher than that for a suburbanite.

To take an example of where flowcharts can lead to trouble, consider a simple rule such as: "The study can be done in the way proposed if the risk is minimal and there is a substantial chance of benefit for the subjects." We could imagine a flowchart with two questions, one about the risk and one about the benefit. Both criteria would have to be met. Now suppose that we quantify risk as the probability of some particular bad event, such as a side effect from an experimental drug, and we quantify benefit as the probability of a good event, such as a cure of a serious disease. Suppose that our judge defines minimal risk as less than 5%, and substantial chance of benefit as more than 20%. This means she would approve a study with 4% risk and 21% chance of benefit, but disapprove a study with 5% risk and 90% chance of benefit.

In contrast, decision analysis would quantify the utilities of the two events. If the disutility of the bad event were, say, four times the utility of the good event, then we would want to approve the study when the probability of the bad event is less than 25% of the probability of the good event. Thus, we would just approve it if the probabilities were, respectively, 5% and 21%, or 20% and 81%, or 0.1% and 0.5%.

It seems arbitrary to set the risk criterion in the same place regardless of the potential benefit. The trouble with categorical rules is that they seem to require this. In real life, people fudge. They let their criterion for minimal risk be influenced by other things they know. So the rule does not help. In fact it hinders, because some judges will want to follow it literally. Thus, the attempt to mechanize judgment fails. People must fall back on trading off quantitative attributes even while trying to follow rules that prohibit such trade-offs.

The utilitarian alternative I advocate is to make the trade-offs and judgments—when they are involved—explicit. Given that judgments are involved anyway, the introduction of judgment is no loss. It is an explicit acknowledgment of what happens anyway. Making the process explicit, in the form of decision analysis, may lead to better judgments. At the very least, explication serves the purpose of describing more accurately how decisions are made, for the benefit of those affected by them. In the next chapter, I begin the discussion of the basis of decision analysis.

The effort to make the trade-offs explicit need not always involve numbers. It could simply involve bearing in mind a rule that permits them. For example, "weigh the probability and magnitude of harm against the benefits." Such a rule, although vague, would be as easy to apply as the (equally vague) rules now in use, but it would also focus judges on the issues that matter most in terms of consequences.

It may seem that decision analysis involves false precision. It is true, of course, that when we judge a probability to be .43, we might actually be happy with a judgment of .38 or .50. Most numerical judgments are soft, and some are softer than others. However, most of the time the results of analysis will not depend on which reasonable numbers we choose. When they do, the decision is truly a close one, and we cannot go *far* wrong with either choice. True precision is not required.

2.5   Conclusion

In this chapter, I have tried to contrast the utilitarian approach I will take with the tradition arising from bioethics as it is practiced. Bioethical practice is concerned with the application of principles. When this practice leads to outcomes that are worse on the whole than could be achieved some other way, we are led to wonder whether we could find a way to achieve better outcomes consistently. Some may say that bad outcomes are just the price of morality, but what is this "morality" that allows us to make things worse for someone else?

A more serious question is whether, perhaps, the principles lead to better outcomes than the direct attempt to get good outcomes. This is an issue I shall address in later chapters. But the general answer is that we can incorporate this possibility into decision analysis itself, as a correction for the possibility of error in the analysis.

The next chapter will go further into the analysis of decisions.

Chapter 3

Utilitarianism and Decision Analysis

This chapter outlines an argument for utilitarianism and the form of decision analysis that is most compatible with it.

3.1 Utilitarianism

Utilitarianism is the view that decisions should maximize the total expected utility of all who are affected. *Utility* is a measure of the value of consequences, a common metric by which the consequences may be compared. A better term would be "good" (Broome 1991). In utilitarianism, when we are faced with two options, we compare them by asking about the difference (positive or negative) between them for each person's good (utility), and then we add up these differences across people. If option 1 is better than option 2 for person A, B, and C by 5 units each but worse for person D by 10 units, then we choose option 1, for a net gain of 5 units. (The units are arbitrary, but the same units must be used for everyone.)

Utilitarianism is very closely related to expected utility theory (EUT), which holds simply that decisions should maximize expected utility, leaving open the question of whose utility is maximized. The expected utility of an option is computed by multiplying the utility of each pos-

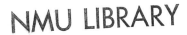

sible consequence by its probability and then adding up these products over all the possible (mutually exclusive) consequences. The probabilities are those of the decision maker, and the utilities are those of whomever the decision is for.

Utilitarianism is similar to—and sometimes identical to—the theory of social welfare in economics. Kaplow and Shavell (2002), for example, use the term "welfare economics" for what is essentially utilitarianism. Economists often question the meaningfulness of interpersonal comparison of utility, so they have developed other forms of welfare economics that do not require such comparison. They doubt that it is possible to say that 5 units of good for me is the same as 5 units for you.

It is worth emphasizing that utilitarianism requires comparison of utility *differences* rather than *levels*. To decide between two options, A and B, you need to know the utility difference between the options for each affected person i, that is $U_i(A) - U_i(B)$. By adding up these differences, some of which may be negative, you find the overall difference between A and B. Although interpersonal comparisons of this sort are sometimes difficult, they are possible in principle and often in fact (Baron 1993a, ch. 5). For some applications, interpersonal comparison is not an important issue. For example, many of the conclusions reached in the law and economics literature do not depend on it. In other cases, such as general policy recommendations, it is often reasonable to assume that each person is represented by the average person. For example, a policy about vaccinations might reasonably assume that people are roughly similar in their utility for the side effects of the vaccine vs. the disease it prevents.

Utilitarianism has provided a controversial approach to decisions about law and policy since its inception. The English term was apparently invented by Jeremy Bentham, a legal reformer. Most of the controversy came (and still comes) from two sources. One is the simplistic and overconfident application of the theory, leading to various bad consequences—that is, errors according to the theory's own standards. (Surely, this problem is not unique to utilitarianism.) The other is the conflict with our moral intuition.

In this chapter, I want to make a few points in favor of utilitarianism as a normative theory. Most of these points are in previous literature (Baron 1993a, 1996a; Broome 1991; Hare 1981; Kaplow and Shavell 2002). Surely, a complete defense of utilitarianism and EUT requires much more than I can say here, but much of it has been said in the references I just cited. The problem I see is that the theory is so often dismissed without a complete understanding. Of course, we can't all take the time to understand every theory before dismissing it, but utilitarianism suffers from a kind a conformity effect, in which everyone thinks that it must be nonsense because everyone else thinks so.[1]

3.1.1 Normative, prescriptive, and descriptive models

Decision theorists distinguish three kinds of models: normative, prescriptive, and descriptive. Failure to make these distinctions leads to spurious criticisms of decision theory and utilitarianism.

Normative theories are standards for evaluation. Psychologists use normative theories to "score" subjects' judgments and decisions. For example, we might ask a subject about a set of choices, and then score them for their internal consistency according to utility theory of some sort.

Descriptive theories describe what people do. Economists call them "positive" theories. Economists often assume that normative and descriptive theories are the same. That is, they assume that people are rational. This is a good working assumption for many purposes, but, in other cases, it misleads us (Baron 2000). Political behavior is such a case, but departures from rationality are found even in markets (Kahneman and Tversky 2000).

Prescriptive theories are prescriptions for what we should do, all things considered, in order to do as well as possible according to the normative standard. A distinction between prescriptive and normative has been implicit in utilitarianism since at least the time of Mill, who argued, in essence, that we ought to honor certain basic liberties—such as free speech—even when we judge that the consequences of doing so would be worse, because such judgments are more often incorrect than correct.

---

[1]Of course some critics of utilitarianism and EUT do read the literature very deeply. To my knowledge, most of their criticisms go against specific forms of each theory, certain ways of developing the theories, or particular assumptions. The problem for the critics is that there are many forms and many ways of defending each form. Moreover, many, if not all, of the specific criticisms can be, and have been, answered. It is an even more formidable task to rebut all the criticisms than it is to criticize all the ways of developing the theories. Most defenders of these theories end up trying to re-state the theory in a clearer and more defensible way, rather than review the massive literature.

The possibility of systematic misjudgment is one of many reasons not to aim to maximize utility in certain situations (Hare 1981). For example, some utilitarians have argued that paternalistic attempts to protect people from bad judgment—such as the failure to let infants' parents decide whether to enroll their dying infants in research—may seem to maximize utility in the case at hand, but the track record of paternalism is sufficiently poor that those who make such attempts should wonder whether they have it right. Prescriptively, it might be better to follow a rule of letting people make decisions, at least in certain types of cases.

The normative-prescriptive distinction blunts the type of criticism that holds that decision theory is impossible or difficult to apply. This is a valid criticism of prescriptive models, but decision theory is normative. The normative-descriptive distinction also blunts the criticism that decision theory disagrees with our intuition. Our intuition may be biased. That is a descriptive question.

The prescriptive-descriptive distinction is not relevant to any questions about normative models, but it is relevant to practical questions about whether people do what they ought to do, and whether they can be helped to make better decisions.

3.1.2 Intuitions and biases

The normative-descriptive distinction is the grist for the psychology of judgment and decisions. We look for systematic biases, or departures from normative models—such as the status-quo effect, in which people regard losses from the status-quo as more serious than gains, even when they are not more serious in fact. Such biases are typically caused by heuristics—that is, rules that people tend to follow out of habit because the rules usually yield acceptable outcomes, such as, "If it ain't broke, don't fix it," or "A bird in the hand is worth two in the bush." The trouble with such rules is that sometimes, if we thought about it, we would see that they lead to worse consequences than the alternative.

As an example, "omission bias" amounts to taking harms of omission less seriously than harms of commission (Ritov and Baron 1990; see also section 9.1.1). For example, failures to prevent diseases through vaccination are often considered less serious than the causing of harm from vaccine side effects. Biases such as this are apparently the basis of philosophical intuitions that are often used as counterexamples to utilitarianism, such as the problem of whether you should kill one person to save five others. Many people feel that they should not kill the one and that, therefore, utilitarianism is incorrect. They assume that their intuitions arise from the moral truth, usually in some obscure way. An alternative view is that intuitions arise from the learning of simple rules that usually coincide with producing good consequences, but, in the critical cases, do not. In terms of consequences, one dead is better than five. Of course, once the intuition starts running, it is bolstered by all sorts of imaginary arguments, some of them about consequences.

3.1.3   Normative theory without intuitions

In this chapter, I am sketching briefly and abstractly one type of argument that can be made for utilitarian decision analysis, an argument that does not depend on our intuitive judgments. The idea that intuitions could serve as the basis of theory came from Chomsky (e.g., 1957), by way of Rawls (e.g., 1971). Chomsky's project was basically psychological. He wanted to use linguistic intuitions to discover our psychological dispositions for language. The parallel inquiry in moral theory or decision theory will discover our psychological dispositions in the same way, but we must have a kind of blind faith in evolution to accept these as the right answer without further justification.

You might wonder how we could develop a normative theory without relying on intuitions. My answer (drawing in a loose way on Popper (1962, particularly the essay on logic and arithmetic) is that we develop an analytic scheme that we impose on the world, and then we reason logically from this scheme. The acceptability of the scheme might depend on intuition of a sort, but it is a different sort from the intuition that tells us not to kill one person in order to save five.

The main analytic scheme for much of decision theory makes distinctions among acts (options), uncertain states of the world, and outcomes or consequences (Savage 1954). Probability is a property of states. Outcomes are determined jointly by acts and states. Good, or utility, is a property of outcomes. My favored version of these theories defines utility as goal achievement, where goals are personal criteria or standards. But the theory could work with other definitions of utility.

Acts and states are distinguished by their controllability. Acts are what we try to decide among.

States and outcomes are both propositions about the world that may be true or false at any given time. Outcomes have value, but states do not. (Insofar as they do, their value is represented in the outcomes.)

Acts and outcomes differ because outcomes are propositions, while acts have no truth value. They follow the logic of imperatives rather than the logic of propositions (Hare 1952). Because outcomes are like states in this regard, outcomes may function as states for other decisions: my decision could create a situation that you then have to deal with as a state of your world.

The act-outcome distinction is important when it comes to distinguishing utilitarian principles from deontological principles. The latter are principles, such as "do no harm directly through action" (but doing harm indirectly through omission is not so bad), or "do not interfere with nature." If we can define "doing harm directly through action" as an outcome, then we could, it seems, incorporate deontological rules into utilitarianism, and utilitarianism would lose its content. Decision theory and utilitarianism assign utilities to outcomes, not to acts. If we assign utilities to types of acts, we can use these to justify rules that violate the spirit of decision theory, which is that decisions should be based on their expected consequences.

Outcomes must be defined as if they were states of the world that need not arise from people's choices. The justification of this restriction is that decision theory is supposed to tell us how to decide about acts. If we incorporate utilities for acts themselves, we incorporate a prejudgment about the answer to the question being asked, the question of what to do. This makes the theory less useful, because it is more circular. To say that an action is bad because it has disutility is to beg the question of why.

This restriction of what counts as an outcome is not as limiting as it might appear to be. If you are bothered by the existence of abortions, then this being bothered is a consequence that you care about. We can thus count your reaction as a consequence for you. If it is stronger than the net benefits of abortion for others in some case, then a utilitarian would say it should not be done.

Although we count your reaction, we do not count your opinion that abortions should not be done, even though this opinion is tightly bound, psychologically, with your reaction. The issue here is how much weight you get in this calculation. Your opinion may be that abortion is really awful, but its effect on your own well-being might be small. If we want to measure your utilities, we have to ask you very carefully, and you have to answer very honestly. In practice, such measurement is difficult. What is important here is that it makes sense in theory. The next section elaborates this issue.

3.1.4   Types of goals: self-interested, moralistic, altruistic, moral

Decisions are designed to achieve goals or, in other words, objectives or values. Goals may be understood as criteria for the evaluation of decisions or their outcomes (Baron 1996a). I use the term *goals* very broadly to include (in some senses) everything a person values.

Goals, in the sense I describe, are criteria for evaluating states of affairs. They are reflectively endorsed. They are the results of thought, and are, in this sense, "constructed," in much the way that concepts are the results of reflection. Goals are not simply desires, and very young children might properly be said to have no goals at all, in the sense at issue.

Your goals fall into four categories: self-interested, altruistic, moralistic, and moral (Baron 2003). These correspond to a two-by-two classification. One dimension of this classification is whether or not your goals depend on the goals of others. The other dimension is whether they concern others' voluntary behavior and their goals for that behavior, or just your own goals and behavior.

	For yourself	For others
Dependent on others' goals	Altruistic	Moral
Independent of others' goals	Self-interested	Moralistic

The idea of dependence on others' goals assumes that goals are associated with the individuals who have them. Your goals are contingent on your existence. If you were never born, no goals would be yours.[2]

---

[2]I do not assume that goals cease with death. Indeed, I have argued that they may continue (Baron 1996a).

Your self-interested goals are those that are yours, in this sense. Altruistic (and moral) goals are goals for the achievement of others' goals. Your altruistic goals concerning X are thus a replica in you of X's goals as they are for X. Altruism may be limited to certain people or certain types of goals, but it rises or falls as the goals of others rise and fall.[3]

We have goals for what other people do voluntarily and for the other goals they have. It is these goals for others that justify laws, social norms, and morality itself. When you have goals for others, you apply criteria to their behavior and goals rather than to your own. But of course these are still your own goals, so you try to do things that affect others' behavior in the most general sense, which includes their goals and all their thinking, as well as their overt behavior (just as self-interested goals may concern your own mental states). And "behavior" excludes involuntary or coerced behavior. When we endorse behavior for others, we want them to want to choose it.

What I call moral goals are goals that others behave so as to achieve each others' goals. These are "moral" in the utilitarian sense only. In fact, they are the fundamental goals that justify the advocacy of utilitarianism (Baron 1996a). I shall return to these goals.

By contrast, moralistic goals are goals for the behavior of others (including their goals) that are independent of the goals of others. People could want others (and themselves) not to clone humans, or not to desire to do it. Often the public discourse about such things is expressed in the language of consequences. Moralistic goals usually come bundled with beliefs that they correspond to better consequences (a phenomenon that has been called "belief overkill" (Jervis 1976; Baron 1998). For example, opponents of human cloning claim that it will demean human life in general. (One could just as easily argue the opposite if cloning is used to cure disease, or even to provide a last-resort means of reproduction.)

In sum, unlike moral goals, moralistic goals can go against the goals of others. When moralistic goals play out in politics, they can interfere with people's achievement of their own goals. That is, if we define "utility" as a measure of goal achievement, they decrease the utility of others.

---

[3]We could imagine negative altruism, in which X wants Y's goals to be frustrated in proportion to their strength. Clearly, such goals exist, but I do not discuss them here.

In bioethics, this seems likely to happen in cases of paternalism: people who make their own decisions are less likely to have moralistic goals imposed upon them.

Moral goals may also involve going against the goals of some in order to achieve the goals of others. But moral goals are those that make this trade-off without bringing in any additional goals of the decision maker regarding the behavior of others.

Altruism and moralism are difficult to distinguish because of the possibility of paternalistic altruism. A true altruist may still act against your stated preferences, because these preferences may depend on false beliefs and thus be unrelated to your true underlying goals (Baron 1996a). Undoubtedly moralists often believe that they are altruists in just this way. However, people think that their values should sometimes be imposed on others even when they (ostensibly) agree that the consequences are worse and that the others involved do not agree with the values being imposed (Baron 2003). Moreover, even when people think that they are being paternalistic and altruistic, they may be incorrect.

Because other people's moralistic goals—in contrast to their altruistic goals and moral goals—are independent of our own individual goals, each of us has reason to want to replace moralistic goals with altruistic goals. Specifically, you will benefit from altruistic and moral goals of others, and you will also benefit from their moralistic goals if these agree with your own goals. But you will suffer from moralistic goals that conflict with your goals. In general, if you are sufficiently concerned about this conflict, you will support greater liberty in individual decision making.

It is conceivable that most moralistic goals have greater benefits than costs, relative to their absence, and that they could not be replaced with other goals—such as moral goals—that had even greater benefits. But it is also conceivable that moralistic goals arise from the same underlying motivation that yields moral goals and that the difference is a matter of belief, which depends on culture, including child rearing and education. Some of the beliefs in question may be false, and subject to correction. To the extent to which moralistic goals can be replaced with more beneficial moral goals, we have reason to try to make this happen. We also have reason not to honor goals that depend on false beliefs (as I discuss in section 3.4).

3.1.5 A norm-endorsement argument

The idea of endorsing norms can provide a way of justifying utilitarianism (Baron 1996a). Norm endorsement is what I call the activity we undertake to try to influence the behavior of others. I have argued that norm endorsement is a fundamental moral activity, in terms of which morality can be defined. What should count as moral, by this view, is what we each have reason to endorse for others and ourselves to follow, assuming that we have put aside our current moral views. By this account, moralistic goals are nonmoral. But we all have reason to endorse moral and altruistic goals. (Specifically, our reasons come from both self-interest and altruism.)

The basis of this argument is an analytic scheme in which we ask about the purpose of moral norms, or, more generally, norms for decision making. The idea is that the act of endorsing norms is fundamental for a certain view of what the question is. There are surely other questions worth answering, but the question of what norms we should endorse for decision making is of sufficient interest, whether or not it exhausts the meaning of "moral" or "rational."

The motivation for norm endorsement can be altruistic, moralistic, or moral. If we want to ask about what norms we should endorse for others, we are concerned about their behavior. Hence, we want to put aside the norms that arise from our current moral and moralistic goals, to see whether we can derive these goals from scratch. Again, this isn't the only question to ask, even within this scheme, but it is a useful question. The answer provides a justification of our goals concerning others' behavior, without the circularity of justifying those goals in terms of goals of the same sort.

Our remaining altruistic goals are sufficient to motivate the endorsement of norms for others' decision making. If we successfully encourage others to rationally pursue their self interest and to be altruistic toward others, they will achieve their own goals better. This will satisfy our own altruism toward them. Note that our altruistic goals concern the achievement of their goals, but we have now used this to justify moral goals, in which we endorse altruistic goals for others.

Consider a society without morality. What this means is that people make no attempt to influence the behavior of others, except as a by-product of attempts to achieve their own self-interested goals. They behave as if they simply have not thought of such a type of behavior as behavior designed to influence others. Thus, they do not engage in political action (unless they are convinced that it is in their narrow self-interest to do so); they do not try to convince others of the correctness of their views about how to behave; they do not instruct their children in any principles except those required for household peace; they do not engage in gossip; and they do not even discuss morality or politics as we know them. This does not mean that people behave badly by our current standards. They still may have a legal system, inherited from an older culture in which the police and courts enforce laws because they are paid to do so. Such a system might survive for a while, since nobody would advocate any change in it. They would still have basic human emotions such as empathy and anger, and they would have altruistic goals, and even a sense of civic duty. They would simply not try explicitly to change each other's behavior in any way. They would be totally tolerant. This might be a relativist's utopia.

Because these people do not try to influence each other, they have no principles or rules about how to do so, if they were to suddenly acquire the idea of doing it. They have no moral principles, no principles for what to do when trying to influence others.

Then, one day, someone thinks of the idea of trying to influence others. Each individual must now decide how to implement this idea, or whether to do so. What would you do in such a situation? What principles would you adopt for this new type of behavior? Why would you engage in it at all?

The reasons would have to come from goals that you already have, other than those goals that we have excluded. If you are going to try to influence the behavior of others who will have no effect on you, perhaps because they will exist after your death, then you must be motivated at least in part by altruism, which is a goal that you already have. It is difficult to think of other goals that might motivate this sort of behavior, except for sadism perhaps, but it is reasonable to assume that pure sadism is weaker than pure altruism.

This would mean that you would have reason to try to influence the behavior of others in ways that will make them more likely to achieve the goals of others. That is all the reason you need to endorse utilitarianism.

You might also have reason to endorse limited forms of utilitarianism, in which the relevant goals to be achieved are those of some group to which you feel loyal. But notice that this feeling of loyalty cannot be based on the moral principles of any group, because these do not exist yet. The problem of whether moral principles should exist if they apply only to limited groups, such as nations or people currently alive, is not peculiar to utilitarianism and is not all that relevant to the issues discussed in this book. The answer often provided is that groups are arbitrary, but this answer may not be sufficient to change the feelings of group loyalty that many people seem to have.

3.1.6   The beginnings of decision analysis

I want to turn now to another topic, before coming back to the rest of what I have to say about utilitarianism in this chapter, namely, decision analysis. *Decision analysis* is a set of prescriptive methods based on utility theory. The ideas grew gradually out of economics, statistics, and psychology in the 1950s and 1960s. This section will discuss one part of decision analysis, the part based on expected utility theory. Then I shall discuss that theory and its relation to utilitarianism.

Decision analysis grew out of statistical decision theory, which had been important in statistics since the early twentieth century. In essence, statistics had been viewed as a decision about whether to accept a hypothesis, given the tolerance for two kinds of errors: accepting a false hypothesis or not accepting a true one. For example, to decide whether a new antiheadache drug was beneficial, you would give the drug to one group of patients, give a placebo (inactive pill) to another group, and then count the number of headaches for each person in both groups. There would be some overlap, but if the drug helps the first group would have fewer headaches on the average.

Statistical decision theory provides rules for the decision to "accept the hypothesis that the drug is effective." The probability that an effect is large enough to be useful can be calculated from the data. The probability depends on the true size of the effect, the number of patients tested, and the length of time of the trial. The cutoff for deciding that the effect is large enough depends on the costs (in utility) of the two errors involved: approving the drug when it really is not effective, and failing to approve it when it is effective. The relative costs of the errors depend on the seriousness of the condition, the availability of other treatment, and the side effects of the drug (and perhaps also its monetary cost).

What developed in the late 1950s and the 1960s, largely because of the efforts of Howard Raiffa (summarized in his 1968 book), was the idea that utility could be assessed and used in a formal way to make decisions. For example, in deciding what probability of guilt should be required for a criminal conviction, we could ask directly, "How bad is a false conviction relative to a false acquittal?" If the answer is 99 times as bad, then we would want the probability of guilt to be 99 times the probability of innocence before we convict someone. That would be a probability of 99%.

Some of the first applications of this idea were in medicine, starting with the seminal article of Ledley and Lusted (1959), in which it was used to decide on treatments for individual patients and for decisions about policies. The year 1968 marked the publication of Howard Raiffa's classic text, *Decision Analysis*.

3.1.7   An example

Figure 3.1 shows a simple example from Behn and Vaupel (1982). The decision is whether to operate on a patient who might have appendicitis. The square box represents a decision, and each circle is a "chance node," a piece of uncertainty that will be resolved. The probabilities of each possible resolution are listed. The probability of appendicitis is p. The two possible outcomes are life and death. We can assign life a utility of 1 and death a utility of 0. To get advice about the decision, we calculate the expected utility of each option. That is, we multiply the probability of getting to each end point on the right times its utility. This gives us the average utility if the same situation were repeated many times. In this case, because death has utility 0, we can ignore the points that end in death. The expected utility of operating is .999 (since the outcome does not depend on whether the patient has appendicitis or not). The expected utility of not operating is $.99 \cdot p + 1 \cdot (1 - p)$. A little algebra shows that, if $p = .1$, then the utilities are equal. Thus, operation is the better decision if $p > .1$ and not operating is better if $p < .1$. If $p = .1$ then the two options are equally good.

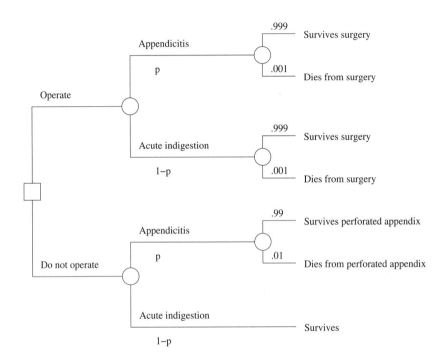

Figure 3.1: Simple decision analysis about appendicitis

This analysis is oversimplified in many ways. It assumes that the probabilities of death from surgery or from a ruptured appendix are known, but the probability of appendicitis is a matter of judgment. In reality, both kinds of probability could be influenced by both statistics about past cases and judgments about the idiosyncrasies of the case at hand. Also, there are only two possible end points, so no deep analysis of utilities is needed. Still, even this simple case shows how decision analysis could yield an informative conclusion about a real situation. This case is just complicated enough that, from looking at the figure, it is not clear what to do. Of course, this is not the only possible analysis of this situation (as Behn and Vaupel show).

A more typical situation would involve outcomes that differed in utility. For example, let us suppose—contrary to fact—that survival after a perforated appendix typically yields a lower quality of life henceforth. If the utility of life in this condition were, say, .9 instead of 1, then we would have to multiply the .99 by .9 instead of by 1.0. This would lower the probability at which operating is neutral, to .009 instead of .1. This is not necessarily obvious from looking at the figure.

Notice that the .9 here represents a kind of goodness that can be taken into account quantitatively—that is, utility. Consider 1,000,000 people in this situation, each with a probability of .009 of having appendicitis. If all had operations, about 1,000 would die from surgery and 999,000 would have normal lives henceforth. If none had operations, 90 would die from a ruptured appendix, 991,000 would live normal lives, and 8,910 would have lives of reduced quality. If these two situations are equally good, then we are trading off the number of lives for quality of life.

Ultimately, we do this. Coronary bypass surgery, for example, has most of its benefit in improving the quality of life, yet it comes with a risk of death from the surgery itself. Implicitly, then, we make this trade-off. Decision analysis makes it more explicit. That is not necessarily always a good thing to do. We can make mistakes with decision analysis, or without it. But the idea of decision analysis is useful for understanding what we are doing when we make any decision.

3.1.8   Expected utility (EU)

The part of decision analysis I have just discussed is based on expected utility theory (EUT). The mathematical and philosophical basis of this theory was developed in the twentieth century (Ramsey 1931; de Finetti 1937; von Neumann and Morgenstern 1947; Savage 1954; Krantz et al. 1970; Wakker 1989), with Savage's 1954 book being the main advance that inspired decision analysis.[4]

EUT can be developed on the basis of another analytic scheme. The scheme involves the distinction among acts (options), uncertain states of the world, and outcomes (Savage 1954). This approach is not so much a substantive view but rather a set of analytic assumptions that we impose on the world. We might do things differently. For example, you might refuse to distinguish options (which you control) and states (which are out of your control) because you think our behavior is determined by the laws of nature and is just like states. Or you might want to assign values to the acts or states themselves. In the latter case, the analysis requires that you simply add this value to all outcomes associated with a given act or state.

Choice 1	State	
Option	A	B
S	$300	$100
T	$420	$0

Choice 2	State	
Option	A	B
U	$500	$100
V	$630	$0

Choice 3	State	
Option	A	B
W	$300	$210
X	$420	$100

Choice 4	State	
Option	A	B
Y	$500	$210
Z	$630	$100

Table 3.1: Four choices illustrating trade-off consistency

Typically, we make a table in which the rows are acts, the columns are states, and the cells are outcomes, such as the choices shown in Table 3.1. In Choice 1, Option S yield $300 if event A happens (e.g., a coin comes up heads) and $100 if B happens. Köbberling and Wakker (2003) consider patterns like those for Choices 1–4. Suppose you are indifferent between S and T in Choice 1, between

---

[4]This subsection may be skipped without loss of continuity, as may any section in this chapter in small print.

U and V in choice 2, and between W and X in Choice 3. Then you ought to be indifferent between Y and Z in Choice 4. Why? Because rational indifference means that the reason for preferring T if A happens, the $120 difference, is just balanced by the reason for preferring S if B happens. Thus, we can say that the difference between $300 and $420 in state B just offsets the difference between $0 and $100 in state A. If you decide in terms of goal achievement, then the 300–420 difference in A achieves your goals (on the whole, taking into account your probability for A) just as much as the $0–$100 difference in B. Similarly, if you are indifferent in Choice 2, then the $500–$630 difference just offsets the same $0–$100 difference. So the $500–$630 difference achieves your goals to the same extent. And if you are indifferent in Choice 3, then the $500–$630 difference in A just offsets the $100–$210 difference in B. So all these differences are equal in terms of goal achievement. In this case, you ought to be indifferent in Choice 4, too. This kind of transitivity, in which Choices 1 through 3 imply the result of Choice 4, plus a couple of other much simpler principles (such as connectedness), *implies expected utility theory.*

The critical idea here is that goals are achieved because of events that happen, not because of events that do not happen. Thus, the difference in goal achievement between outcomes in State A cannot be affected by the difference in State B, because the states are mutually exclusive.

Note that we are also assuming that the idea of differences in goal achievement is meaningful. But it must be meaningful if we are to make such choices at all in terms of goal achievement. For example, if States A and B are equally likely, then any choice between S and T must depend on which difference is larger, the difference between the outcomes in A (which favor option T) or the difference between the outcomes in B (which favor S). It makes sense to say that the difference between $200 to $310 has as much of an effect on the achievement of your goals as the difference between $0 and $100.

3.1.9   Individual and group

Utilitarianism is closely related to EU theory. When a group of people all face the same decision, then the two models clearly dictate the same choice. For example, suppose each of 1,000 people faces a 0.2 probability of some disease without vaccination, but the vaccine causes an equally serious disease with a probability of 0.1. The best decision for each person is to get the vaccine. If everyone gets the vaccine, then we expect that 100 will get the disease caused by the vaccine, instead of 200 getting the other disease. This is what utilitarianism would recommend.

The relationship goes deeper than this. It is possible to show that, if the utility of each person is defined by EU, then, with some very simple assumptions, the overall good of everyone is a sum of individual utilities (Broome 1991). In particular, we need to assume the "Principle of Personal Good" (Broome 1991, p. 165): "(a) Two alternatives are equally good if they are equally good for each person. And (b) if one alternative is at least as good as another for everyone and definitely better for someone, it is better."[5]

To make this argument, Broome (1991) considers a table such as the following. Each column represents a state of nature. Each row represents a person. There are s states and h people. The entries in each cell represent the utilities for the outcome for each person in each state. For example u_{12} is the utility for Person 1 in State 2.

$$
\begin{array}{cccc}
u_{11} & u_{12} & \ldots & u_{1s} \\
u_{21} & u_{22} & \ldots & u_{2s} \\
\cdot & \cdot & \ldots & \cdot \\
\cdot & \cdot & \ldots & \cdot \\
u_{h1} & u_{h2} & \ldots & u_{hs}
\end{array}
$$

The basic argument, in very broad outline, shows that total utility is an increasing function of both the row and column utilities, and that the function is additive for both rows and columns. EU theory implies additivity for each row. For a given column, the Principle of Personal Good implies that the utility for each column is an increasing function of the utilities for the individuals in that column. An increase in one entry in the cell has to have the same effect on both the rows and the columns, so the columns must be additive too. [6]

Some have argued that social welfare must take into account properties of the distribution of utility, not just utility. For example, some think that it is more important to maximize the well being of the poorest people than to maximize total utility (e.g., Rawls 1971). Greene and Baron (2001) have argued that this view is the result of an intuitive rule that is

---

[5]This is a variant of the basic idea of "Pareto optimality." This variant assumes that the probabilities of the states do not depend on the person. It is as though the theory were designed for decision makers with their own probabilities.

[6]For details, see Broome 1991, particularly, pp. 68, 69, and 202.

valid when applied to ordinary goods, such as money. Indeed, we can do more good by giving $100 to a poor person than by giving $100 to a rich person, but this is (arguably) because the money has more utility to the poor person—that is, does more good. But an equal amount of *utility* is by definition just as much good for either person. Yet, people treat utility like money, and this intuition results in judgments that are internally inconsistent (Greene and Baron 2001).

Similarly, the use of different utilities for social and individual welfare calculations can result in decisions that maximize social welfare yet make each person worse off. For example, suppose that each person rationally considers a 50% chance to win $300 as better than $100 for sure. But a social welfare theorist might take ex-post inequality into account and, noticing that the same gamble played for everyone would leave half the people with $300 (plus their current wealth) and half with nothing. A judgment of the ultimate social welfare would declare that it would be socially better to give $100 to everyone, thus leading to the worse of two choices for each person. Kaplow and Shavell (2002) use this kind of argument against all sorts of principles of fairness that go against utility maximization. They point out two possibilities. One: fairness principles agree with utility maximization. Or two:, it is possible to have a situation in which the application of a fairness principle makes everyone worse off from each person's individual point of view (in particular, when everyone is in the same situation). Of course, these situations are highly hypothetical, but, as Kaplow and Shavell point out, a normative theory should apply everywhere, even to hypothetical situations.

3.2 Intuitive judgments

If utilitarianism is so great, one might ask, why do our intuitions so often disagree with it? Perhaps because they often agree, in fact. Moral intuitions may develop in response to observations that certain types of behavior lead to certain types of consequences. Like children's theories about science and mathematics, these observations might be reasonable first approximations, yet not quite accurate. They may be overgeneralizations, of a sort.

3.2.1   Intuitions as overgeneralizations

For example, when children learn the meanings of words such as "doggie," they often apply the term to cats or hamsters. A little later, when faced with arrays like the following,

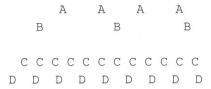

they say that there are more Ds than Cs, responding to the length of the two rows rather than the number. While they correctly acknowledge that the D row is longer than the C row, and that the the A row has more letters than the B row, they mistakenly say that the A row is longer than the B row. In essence, they conflate length and number, failing to distinguish them, much as younger children fail to distinguish cats and dogs. When they learn that the B row is in fact longer than the A row, they often come to assert that it also has more letters (Lawson, Baron, and Siegel 1974; Baron, Lawson, and Siegel 1975).

When they are somewhat older, they learn to compute the area of a parallelogram by multiplying the base times the height. Some children then apply the same formula to a trapezoid (Wertheimer 1959). All three of these examples can be seen as cases of overgeneralization. A rule is learned that works in one case because it is correlated with the correct rule. It is overgeneralized to a case in which the correlation is broken. Of course, every case of overgeneralization is accompanied by a case of undergeneralization. If an incorrect rule is applied, then a correct rule is not applied, perhaps because it isn't known at all. It might be more appropriate to call these cases of misgeneralization rather than overgeneralization, but it is the latter that we see.

Another way of describing the situation is that people have too few rules. In the case of dogs and cats, length and number, or parallelograms and trapezoids, people use one rule when they should use two. (Later I shall argue that, in some cases, the problem is exactly the opposite from what it seems to be—that is, people have many rules when one would do.)

Misgeneralization can be prevented through an understanding of the purpose of rules. The idea of area is a useful concept with all sorts of purposes, such as predicting the amount of paint needed to cover something, the amount of cloth needed to make it, its weight (with a constant thickness), and so on. To serve these purposes, area must have certain properties, such as being conserved over transformations of cutting and moving pieces. Students can, in principle, use their knowledge of purposes to correct misunderstandings of rules, such as the rule for the area of the parallelogram. Similarly, concepts of length and number have purposes, and these purposes are not well served if counting becomes a way of judging length, for example.

The same kinds of psychological mechanisms affect our intuitions about policy. By intuitions, I mean our judgments of better and worse, of the sort that come to mind without any analysis. These intuitions can be studied in psychology experiments, and their effect can be seen in the policy world itself. When the experiments show phenomena that parallel what we observe in the real world of policy, we gain confidence that the same psychological mechanisms are involved. We can never be certain, but psychology experiments can provide us with additional evidence, perhaps enough to take action.

3.2.2   Intuitive judgments as prescriptive rules

Although intuitive rules can arise from misgeneralization and failure to consider purposes, they can also arise as purposive shortcuts, designed intentionally, or adapted unintentionally, to save time in thinking while doing a reasonably good job. Perhaps an example is a heuristic I use, partly because I have always used it without thinking, but partly because, when I think about it, it seems reasonable to keep using. Specifically, when I teach a large class, I try to follow rigid rules for grading, with the rules announced in advance to all students. This saves me time, and it reduces disputes with students. Given that the assignment of grades is surely full of errors anyway, it isn't clear that further thinking would do much good anyway.

Hare (1981) argues that strict utilitarians can follow rigid rules. They must believe that their attempts to calculate utilities in each case are sufficiently error prone so that any given conclusion in favor of rule violation is likely to be incorrect. Even though there are surely cases in which we should not follow the rule, we are incapable of recognizing them with sufficient accuracy. For example, we might argue against active euthanasia on these grounds: we would grant that it is justified in some cases but doubt anyone's ability to recognize these cases correctly.

Now, this is a nice argument in principle, but note that the same argument can be applied to the following simplistic utilitarian rule: "Do whatever seems to do the most good." Surely *this* rule will lead to worse consequences on occasion than some other rule (varying from case to case). I suspect we cannot recognize the exceptions well enough to confidently violate this simplistic rule, but I can't prove my case.

3.3   Multiattribute utility theory (MAUT)

A second type of decision analysis, other than that based on EU theory, is based on the idea that utility itself could be analyzed into attributes or components. This was part of the economic theory of the consumer, which saw the various goods and services consumed as components of a larger "bundle." The theory has been applied to attributes of individual consumer goods, such as price and quality. (And quality itself could be decomposed further, as done in *Consumer Reports* magazine.)

Again, Raiffa had the idea of measuring these utilities directly. With Ralph Keeney, he developed specific methods for measuring utilities, some based on EU theory (Keeney and Raiffa 1976/1993). The theory behind this type of decision analysis is multiattribute utility theory, or MAUT. The theory is implemented in a variety of ways in practice, perhaps the most useful being called "conjoint analysis," a term derived from "conjoint measurement," which is the theoretical basis for MAUT (Krantz et al. 1971; see Baron 2000, ch. 14, for an introduction).

As an example, consider a decision about which of several drugs to take for pain reduction for a condition expected to last for several months. The drugs differ in daily cost, effectiveness in reducing pain, side effects, and potential for addiction. We will assume that the total utility of each drug is the sum of its utilities on each of these dimensions.

In order for this assumption to hold, the utilities on the dimensions must be independent. In other words, the effect of each dimension on the total utility must be the same, regardless of the levels of the other dimensions. Reduction of pain by a certain amount must be valued just as much, for its own sake, regardless of the price, for example. We can test this assumption in various ways, but the simplest is just to imagine how the level of one dimension might affect the relative utility of two others. In particular, we want to make sure that the trade-off between two dimensions does not depend on the level of a third dimension.

A possible example is that potential for addiction might affect the utility of cost relative to pain reduction. If you get addicted, you might have to take the drug for a longer period of time (perhaps cutting down gradually). This might mean that you would have to pay more in total. Because of this, you would not be willing to pay as much per day for a given level of pain reduction.

In an analysis, you might solve this problem by using expected total cost as the relevant dimension, rather than daily cost. Thus, even when dimensions are not initially independent, you can sometimes redefine them so that they are (Keeney 1992).

The basic idea is to use some sort of judgment task to assign a utility to each level of each attribute, and then add the utilities for each drug to get a total. In principle, you could get the utilities through direct judgments. You could define some difference along one dimension as the basic unit of utility and then compare everything to that. For example, you could define the difference between no pain reduction and total pain reduction as one unit. Then you might ask, "How much am I willing to pay per day for total pain reduction?" Suppose it is $50. Then you can say that the difference between $0 and $50 is also one unit of utility. Because the dimensions are independent (assuming that they are), you can be sure that a change from $0 to $50 will just compensate for a change from no pain reduction to total pain reduction.

Other kinds of judgments might involve proportions. You could, for example, judge that the utility of the difference between $10 and $20 per day is one twentieth of the utility of the difference between no pain reduction and complete reduction. Note that the utility scale for each dimension need not be a linear function of the measure of that dimension. In the example just given, the utility difference between $10 and $20 is one twentieth of the utility difference between $0 and $50. This would make sense if you become more sensitive to price, the more you pay, so that the difference between \$40 and \$50 would represent a greater utility difference than that between \$10 and \$20.

In practical applications of methods such as these, it is often convenient to assume that the utility functions within each dimension are approximately the same for everyone. For example, if the disutility of price is an upwardly curved function of price, we could assume the same function for everyone. The errors that result from violations of this assumption are usually small. Where people differ is in the relative weight that they place on each dimension. Rich people (or people covered by insurance), for example, might care a lot more about pain reduction than price, relative to the weight that others place on these dimensions. Thus, in carrying out decision analysis, it is often sufficient to elicit relative weights of dimensions, and then get the functions within each dimension from just a few subjects on the assumption that they will be the same. For this reason, many decision analysts use a "dimension utility" that is distinct from the actual utility. To get the actual utility from the dimension utility, we multiply the latter by the weight of the dimension for the person.

The simplest method for eliciting utilities for an individual subject does not require this method of dimension weights. It is to present a subject with objects that vary in the levels of the dimensions and ask for an overall rating of each on a one to seven scale, for example. We could present a series of hypothetical drugs varying in price, effectiveness, side effects, and addictiveness. All that is required is to assume that drugs with the same rating have the same overall utility. For example, if drug A had a cost of \$50 and 100% effectiveness and drug B had a cost of \$0 and 0% effectiveness, and the two drugs were the same in other dimensions, they should get the same rating. In actual practice, the procedure allows for error and tries to develop a set of utilities that yield the smallest error in explaining the ratings. (See Baron 2000, for a somewhat more thorough introduction.)

3.4   Attributes and values

The attributes in a multiattribute analysis usually correspond to separate goals, objectives, or values, terms I shall use interchangeably. These values are criteria for evaluating outcomes or states of affairs. We can judge a given state in terms of the extent to which it achieves a goal or objective, or satisfies a value. These values matter to the decision maker. They are his criteria, not someone else's. Thus, it makes sense to let these values define his utility. That is the point, and, if the values do not serve this purpose, then they are incorrect. And if the utility derived from them does not define a person's good, likewise, something is wrong.

Keeney (1992) makes an important distinction between *fundamental values* and *means values*, to which I refer frequently. A means value is valued because it is a means to a fundamental value. A person trying to lose weight will value Diet Coke because she believes that it will help her lose weight. If she learns that it does not (e.g., because it only increases the craving for real sugar), then she will not value it anymore. The goal of losing weight might also be a means to better health. Then it, too, is a means value. But if the purpose is to look better, and if her judgment is that losing weight is inherently part of that, then it is not a means value but a fundamental value.

The difference is that fundamental values cannot be changed by changing beliefs (at least not immediately). Means values are related to fundamental values through beliefs about the extent to which the means value helps to satisfy fundamental values. If the beliefs change, then the means value changes immediately.

The difference is important because fundamental values represent a person's true good, but means values do not necessarily do that, because the beliefs that serve them could be incorrect. If I know that you want to lose weight, and I also know that Diet Coke does not help, despite the fact that you think it does, then I do not help you achieve your true goal by getting you to drink more of it. More generally, means values based on false beliefs should not be part of a person's utility (Baron 1996a).

Of course, such hypothetical examples are unrealistic, because it would be easy for me to change your belief. But it is not always so easy to do that. We still then are faced with decisions that affect others, in which we can do what they believe serves their fundamental values or what we believe serves them. If we are sure of our belief, then we do more good by following it.

This puts aside the true goal that others might have of having their wishes followed. People may desire such autonomy for its own sake, as a fundamental value. But that value, while it must be counted, may conflict with other values that they have, so we may still do more good by overriding their value for autonomy, or not.

3.5 Conclusion

This chapter has presented a brief introduction to an alternative approach to problems in bioethics, based on analysis of consequences of decisions. In subsequent chapters, I shall provide further examples, which I hope will clarify and illustrate the features of utility theory.

Often, in practice, the theory cannot yield a definitive answer because relevant facts are unknown. That isn't quite right. Really, we should always be able to apply EU theory by quantifying our uncertainty with probabilities. A better way to put it is that, in many situations, our decision could change when new knowledge becomes available.

Of course, quantification has its problems. In addition to the problem of imprecision—which I have argued is either irrelevant or inconsequential (because decisions that hinge on precision are close ones)—we have the problem that the utilities we try to measure are often unavailable. I have argued that values and goals are constructed, in the way that concepts are. But this does not prevent them from being real and fairly stable. If we sample the utilities of some population of people, we are likely to get a reasonable, if imprecise, average measure.

It is also true that our methods for measuring utility are crude. When time was first invented as a measurable quantity, the methods of measurement were biased (in the way in which sundials are sensitive to the season) and crude. That is our current state of knowledge of utility measurement (Baron 2000). But utility, like time, can become a better-defined construct as we learn how to measure it better.

Despite these problems, utility theory is often able to locate the source of the problem in a way that focuses on consequences. Once we see that both sides of a controversy can point to some outcome that is better if they prevail, we can see just where they differ. We can often make a quantitative judgment that will settle the question, at least to our own satisfaction.

The next chapter illustrates some of the trade-offs that involve new technologies, which are often a cause of concern in bioethical writing.

Chapter 4

Going Against Nature

Ask most citizens for examples of issues in bioethics, and they tend to think of cases in which people try to "play God"—that is, to manipulate nature. These include genetic engineering of crops, cloning for human reproduction, and using new technologies to make "designer babies," to increase the human lifespan, to rid people of undesirable traits such as aggression, and to improve mental function (Farah 2002). A recent report of the President's Council on Bioethics (2003) notes (in ch. 1), "Precisely because the new knowledge and the new powers impinge directly upon the human person, and in ways that may affect our very humanity, a certain vague disquiet hovers over the entire enterprise."

The idea that it is morally wrong to go against nature is surely very old. It is a traditional part of Catholic moral theology (Finnis 1980). Many philosophers, most notably David Hume, have argued that "is" cannot imply "ought." The facts of nature are what "is." To conclude anything from these facts about what we should do requires an additional premise, a general principle that it is wrong to go against nature. The attempt to make the argument without this premise stated explicitly is the "naturalistic fallacy." An example is, "Women evolved to care for children; therefore, they should not work outside the home." When people attempt to state the missing premise, they run into trouble. It is difficult to define what is "natural" in a way that excludes in-vitro fertilization but includes airplanes and telephones. (Finnis 1980 provides the best effort I have seen.)

Utilitarians do not accept arguments from nature as a premise. Indeed, Richard Hare's arguments (1952, 1963, 1981) about the logic of moral terms stand at the center of modern utilitarianism. However, we can understand some of the opposition to going against nature in terms of various heuristic or intuitive principles, which are generally good rules of thumb. Careful utilitarian analysis of decisions involving nature requires us to separate what matters, in terms of consequences, from intuitions that do not apply to the case at hand. This chapter explores some of these issues.

The intuitions are strong. Many new technologies and new ideas arouse a "yuck reaction," a feeling of disgust, which often drives moral judgment (for example, Haidt and Hersh 2001).

4.1   Enhancements: genes, drugs, and mind control

Much of the recent literature on bioethics, both popular and academic, has concerned the legitimacy of various technological enhancements. It is one thing, the story goes, to use technology to cure disease and disability. It is quite another to use technology to make people better. The examples run the gamut from mundane to fantastic science fiction. Among the mundane examples are hair dye, baldness remedies, exercise and diet for body image (as distinct from health), cosmetics, corsets (no longer in fashion, it seems), coffee for alertness, higher education (for enriching life), human-potential classes, and meditation. At the other end we have gene therapy to raise intelligence, drugs to increase longevity, drugs to improve mood, and eugenics through selective breeding, artificial insemination, or direct genetic manipulation. In between are Ritalin and Prozac—drugs that have clear uses in curing disorders but also may be used to improve mood and performance in people who are not ill or disordered by the usual criteria—liposuction, botox, and breast implants to increase breast size.

The objections raised are of many sorts. One is that these tools could become widely used, or permanent and irreversible (as in the case of eugenics) and change human nature. Presumably that is a bad thing, but I have just argued that it is irrelevant. Another is that they will create inequality because they will not be available to all. Still, another is that they are misuses of the technologies in question.

To begin with, it seems that some of the objections are inconsistent at least. Drugs are considered inappropriate as mood enhancers, but watching Marx Brothers movies is appropriate. What is the difference? Are drugs "artificial?" Mood enhancing drugs and humorous fiction have both been around since before history.

Perhaps one issue is that good things must be paid for, if only through a proper attitude of involvement (of the sort required to appreciate a movie). It is acceptable to seek enlightenment by study with a guru but not by taking LSD. If good things were free, what would motivate people to work? Clearly this line of argument does not go very far by itself. Many of the good things in life are free and available to all.

Another issue is addiction. If mood altering drugs are too easily available, people might all become hippies, grooving on nature, not doing any work. This may be a problem, but it is not a problem with Ritalin and Prozac, which are taken more to enhance work than to replace it.

What are the real dangers? Let us look at these new technologies from the perspective of consequences. Indeed, many of the standard objections can be restated in these terms.

4.1.1   Risk

Many new technologies are in fact risky, both in the short run and the long run. Drugs have side effects. Eugenics could eliminate genes that have benefits yet unknown, which might emerge in a different environment. (The same gene that causes sickle-cell disease also makes people resistant to malaria.)

In the face of such risks, some writers and governmental bodies (in particular, the European Union) have advocated a "precautionary principle," in which new technologies are not adopted unless they are known to be risk free. As other writers have noted (Foster and Vecchia 2002–2003; Sunstein 2003; Wiener 2001), such a principle would paralyze us if we took it seriously. Decision analysis tells us to weigh expected risks against expected benefit.

Can we do this, though? So many technologies have had unforeseen side effects that emerged months or years after the technologies were adopted. Approved drugs have been recalled. Thalidomide was approved in Europe, and its widespread use as an antinausea drug for pregnant women led to thousands of serious birth defects. (It was not approved in the United States, in fact.) Asbestos was widely installed in buildings as a safety measure against fire, and now people are spending billions of dollars to remove it. (Much of it is not, in fact, so risky.) Once-beneficial technologies, such as atomic energy, are now seen as military dangers. Are the benefits of the automobile worth the costs in pollution and global warming? Perhaps, but it isn't obvious.

On the other hand, most economic analyses indicate that technology is the driving force of progress. The examples just listed are in the minority. If we lower our risk threshold so that drugs such as Thalidomide are never approved, we will fail to approve many other drugs with benefits that outweigh their risks and costs. We will prevent harm through action and through change in the status quo, but we will cause much greater harm through inaction.

Decision analysis, in the form of risk analysis, can provide the best possible compromise. Decision analysis usually estimates probabilities by using expert judgments. These are surely better than nothing, or better than some vague "precautionary principle." But it can do still better. In particular, decision analysis can build in corrections for its own uncertainty.

Most decision analysis textbooks advocate "sensitivity analysis." This amounts to asking whether the result—the recommended option—would change if various elements of the analysis were changed. For example, would we still recommend approval of the drug if the probability of serious side effects were twice our best estimate? To do this sort of analysis, we simply run through the analysis several times with the numbers changed. This is instructive, but it is not what I mean.

Rather, I prefer to taking a population view of the estimates themselves. We have real data on the validity of such estimates. We can compare expert judgments of the probability of events with the occurrence of the events themselves. Mathematically, we plot a graph in which the probability estimate is on the abscissa (horizontal axis) and the occurrence or nonoccurrence of the event is on the ordinate. Of course, these points will be 1 when the event happens and 0 when it does not. Then, as shown hypothetically in Figure 4.1, we fit a best-fitting line to the points—that is, a line that comes as close as possible to all the points in vertical position.[1] We can then use this best-fitting line to correct expert judgments. On the basis of previous literature, we would expect the true probability of a bad event to be higher than predicted when the prediction is very low. This is a way of including a "precautionary principle" of a different sort.

For example, suppose our graph tells us that when experts estimate that the probability of unforeseen side effects that are serious enough to change the recommendation for a drug is .01, the actual frequency of such an event is .03, we simply substitute .03 for .01 when we do our decision analysis with a new drug. This is the best we can do. (Henrion and Fischhoff [1986] compared the probabilities given by physicists in estimating basic physical constants with the "true" [most recent] values, finding fairly substantial overconfidence of this sort.)

This approach is a mathematical embodiment of a general utilitarian principle, which is to take into account the possibility of our own error when we estimate which option maximizes expected utility. The classic examples are political terrorism and adultery. People who commit such acts often think that they are for the best, imagining the few cases in which they were (e.g., *Lady Chatterly's Lover*, for adultery). But, if they consider the facts that almost all terrorists and adulterers have had the same thoughts and that almost all of these have been incorrect, they would realize that their best utilitarian judgment would be to avoid the act in question.

The President's Council on Bioethics (2003) raises another issue about risk balancing, in the case of "designer babies." Who should decide? In particular, when should parents be able to take risks for their unborn child, in the hopes of having a superior child? Surely, when decisions are made by individuals rather than government regulators, there will be more errors that result merely from individual variation in decision-making competence, as well as random variation in competence within each individual. As I shall discuss in other cases, there is a trade-off here between these increased errors on one side and these three factors on the other side: the educational benefits (for improved decision making)

---

[1]More precisely, the line is chosen to minimize the sum of the squares of the vertical distance between the line and each point.

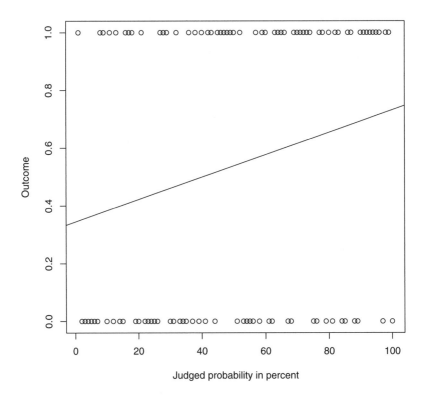

Figure 4.1: Occurrence or nonoccurrence as a function of judged probability.

of autonomy in decision making; the failure of blanket regulations to adapt to individual differences (assuming that individuals can do better at this); and the very real possibility of regulatory error, which may render regulation not all that much better, as its most idealistic proponents might hope. Which side should win is, as usual, an empirical question. In the absence of data, we must make our best guess.

4.1.2 Inequality

The President's Council on Bioethics (2003) also points out that use of technology can lead to increased inequality if it ends up helping those who can pay and does not help those who cannot pay.

Utilitarians have two reasons to oppose inequality. First, a more equal distribution of certain goods, particularly money, might increase total utility, assuming that the total of the goods does not decrease too much as a result of redistribution. This is because utility for many goods, especially money, is marginally declining. A given amount of money—for example, $1,000, means a lot more to a poor farmer in Togo than it does to Bill Gates. In the case of money, people usually spend money on things that do more to achieve their goals before they spend it on other things. The farmer will buy things that are essential to his and his family's survival. Bill Gates (if he doesn't give it to the farmer through a charity) might take his family out to dinner—in Paris.

Second, inequality creates envy in those who lose out. This is more difficult because we might want to discourage envy by ignoring it in our calculations.

The first reason is irrelevant to the case in which the only option is whether to help some or do nothing so as to maintain equality. The classic case (foreshadowed in the Talmud and elsewhere) is *Sophie's Choice* (the novel by William Styron, subsequently made into a movie), in which Sophie had to decide whether to save one of her children from death in a concentration camp—or neither. She chose one, and felt guilty about having to decide. But, from a utilitarian perspective, she did the right thing at the time.

The second reason may be more relevant. But, in fact, the options considered so far are not the only ones. Governments have the power to redistribute income. If inequality is so great that envy is reducing total utility, then governments have the option to reduce the envy by taking from the rich and giving to the poor. This is a decision that is independent of the decision to allow an additional good that might benefit the rich more because they can pay for it.

By analogy, if government should prohibit biotechnological improvements on the grounds that only some could afford them, then perhaps it should also prohibit $100,000 automobiles and $10,000,000 houses. (I discuss this possibility in section 4.1.4.)

4.1.3   Positional goods

Behind some of the objections is another point that can be included in a decision analysis of expected consequences. Suppose a drug is invented that increases our height. It has no side effects but it costs a couple of thousand dollars. Taller people do better at most things on the average, including making money and getting elected to public office. Knowing this, people will take the drug so that each of them can be taller. But notice that only relative height is valuable, not absolute height. An increase in the number of tall people will not increase average income, nor the number of elected officials. At worst, everyone will feel that they must shell out $2,000 in order not to fall behind. Height is a "positional good" (Hirsch 1976).

Many of the personal qualities that biotechnology could enhance are partly positional. Physical beauty or attractiveness is desired in part because of its advantages in competition for mates, jobs, and advancement. To the extent to which competition is involved, it is positional. But one might argue that it is simply more pleasant to live in a world full of attractive people than a world full of ugly ones, so attractiveness has a positive externality. It may even have benefits for the person in terms of positive self-regard, in an absolute sense rather than a competitive sense. Intelligence is similar, in that high intelligence gives people a competitive advantage but also has personal and social value of its own.

The possibility that the effects of intervention are positional adds an additional requirement to the measurement of values in decision analysis. When we measure the value of being taller, thinner, or smarter by asking hypothetical questions, we must ask people how this value depends on their relative position. So, for example, we should ask people,

"What is the value to you of a pill that would increase your IQ by 10 points if the average stays at 100?" and also "What is your part of the value of a pill that would increase everyone's IQ by 10 points?" The first question includes the competitive value, and the second does not. We could imagine questions in between, such as, "What is the value of a pill that will increase your IQ by 10 points, if 50% take the same pill?" In this way, we can estimate what part of the value is positional and what part is "real."

Armed with this information, we then need to estimate, given the cost of the IQ pill, how many will buy it in a steady state, and then use the hypothetical questions to estimate its value for that number. Of course, it is more complicated because the price will come down over time, and more people will buy it.

Positional goods have a darker side. What about those who cannot afford the pill? They will suffer a utility loss with each new person who takes it, because they will lose competitively. We can estimate this effect, too, by asking people about their negative value for an IQ pill that was effective for others but not for them (for different proportions of others). Given what we know about the greater utility effect of losses than of gains, it might turn out that the IQ pill would be a bad deal on the whole, despite its positive externalities and benefits to those who take it. Or it might still be beneficial on the whole.

This is a potentially answerable question, not a deep mystery. The problems of probability and utility estimation are simply problems. Certainly, we could make errors in these tasks, but that is true of any method of decision making.

4.1.4   Waste

Cosmetic surgery seems like a wasteful luxury when so many people in the world cannot see a doctor or nurse even when they are gravely ill. We thus object to some medical technologies because it is greedy to use them. The use of whole-body scans to detect cancer is another example. The money could be spent much more cost-effectively (e.g., on treating AIDS in Africa), even though it may do some good.

It is difficult to include this issue in a decision analysis, in part because all the relevant options are not on the table. The rich who pay for cosmetic surgery and other fancy procedures might put their money to better use by giving it to charity or investing it. But they have already, in some sense, made their decisions about how much to invest or give away.

Arguably, it is not the job of medical decision analysis or bioethics to influence people's choices among consumption, savings, and charity. Rather, that is the job of the tax system and other economic instruments. Even exhortation from clerics and others about giving more to charity need not be given in the context of a particular medical decision.

The tax system is almost ideal for reducing waste in consumptions. One traditional mechanism is a luxury tax. But this tax requires the government to decide what is a luxury and what is wasteful. Perhaps the government could do this, but another way is surely easier to implement and possibly more accurate. This is a graduated consumption tax such as that proposed by Edward McCaffery (2002). People pay an increasing amount of tax on their consumption. The first $20,000 of consumption might be free of tax in the United States on the grounds that it is required for "necessities." Luxuries are what you buy when you have satisfied your basic needs. The more you spend, the less utility you get per dollar. If this is not true, you are not spending wisely. You should make sure to buy the things that give you the greatest utility per dollar. Thus, there is little utility loss from discouraging spending beyond a certain annual amount per person through the tax system, because little utility is gained from the spending. Because there is little utility loss, this is also the most painless way to impose taxes. Note that, under this plan, money that is earned but saved is not taxed until it is withdrawn from savings and spent. This makes sense because the utility of saving is more nearly linear. Saving benefits both the saver, in the long run, and others, through investment.

McCaffery has argued that ordinary medical expenses should be tax free. He would tax the kinds of extraordinary procedures under discussion here. The idea of making ordinary medical expenses tax free is that they are more difficult to control, or, put another way, for those who need them, they have very high utility per dollar. This proposal gets the government back into the business of deciding what is a luxury. An alternative to McCaffery's proposal is to require everyone to have medical insurance (if necessary with a subsidy for the poor). The insurance would cover these ordinary expenses beyond a certain amount per year, so that only the insurance premium would fall under the consumption tax. Insurance companies would then have to decide what they would cover, but this is another issue. In principle, different plans could have different coverages for luxury medical care.

More generally, what is bad about luxury medical care, insofar as its badness is the result of its being a luxury, is the same thing that is bad about all luxuries. It is most efficient to treat them together. If we prohibit luxury A and allow luxury B, then we lose total utility. People would be buying B, even though they would get more utility per dollar from A. By allowing but discouraging both, we would allow people to spend their limited luxury dollars so that each person gains the most.

Like many economic arguments, the one I have just made is utopian. What should we do in the meantime? Might it be better to ban or discourage certain luxuries now, while waiting for utopia to arrive? For example, what if we taxed medical luxuries and used the proceeds to help pay for medical care for the poor? Or what if we just prohibit them on the grounds that doctors have better things to do with their limited time?

Both of these solutions might be better than nothing, but they both have the political disadvantage of making people feel that utopia isn't needed. (For the same reason, Karl Marx did not give money to beggars, he said.) Moreover, the benefits are much more limited than those of the utopian solution. If we tax medical luxuries only, people will simply buy other luxuries that give them less utility per dollar. They will not save much more or give much more to charity. If we outlaw cosmetic surgery (or something more luxurious that doesn't exist yet), then people who would have become cosmetic surgeons will not necessarily go in for emergency medicine instead. They might become tax lawyers (assuming that this is another luxury occupation).

In sum, the problem of waste is a real problem, but not one that we can do much about if all we can control are medical decisions. If we realize this, we can put aside this objection when we consider why new technology should be regulated. But we might tax unusually high consumption.

4.1.5   Buttressing beliefs

More generally, many of the concerns that critics have about biotechnology have a utilitarian reflection. They do affect consequences. Other concerns are more difficult to express in these terms, but not impossible. For example, some critics of biotechnology say that it is overreaching, like greed. This is a criticism based on the motive rather than the decision or the result. Perhaps the encouragement of biotechnology also encourages bad motives. This is a consequence. It is, to me, far-fetched, although eloquent writers can make it seem more compelling.

Other concerns seem more fanciful, almost designed to buttress a conclusion already formed. For example, the President's Council on Bioethics (2003, ch. 2) argues against designer babies: "This leads to the question of what it might mean for a child to live with a chosen genotype: he may feel grateful to his parents for having gone to such trouble to spare him the burden of various genetic defects; but he might also have to deal with the sense that he is not just a gift born of his parents' love but also, in some degree, a product of their will." Applied bioethics writing often talks in terms of "questions" rather than answers, but the answer is implied that this is a problem. It is, of course, a question what it might mean, but it is difficult to imagine that it would so consistently mean something negative so that government should prevent it on these grounds. Only a very intrusive, one might say communist, government would be so confident.

Still other arguments represent the naturalistic fallacy: It is so, so it should be so. For example, arguing against attempts to influence reproduction (President's Council on Bioethics 2003, ch. 2): "The salient fact about human procreation in its natural context is that children are not made but begotten. By this we mean that children are the issue of our love, not the product of our wills. A man and a woman do not produce or choose a particular child, as they might buy a particular brand of soap; rather, they stand in relation to their child as recipients of a gift. Gifts and blessings we learn to accept as gratefully as we can; products of our wills we try to shape in accordance with our wants and desires. Procreation as traditionally understood invites acceptance, not reshaping or engineering." Yes. But what is wrong with changing this to some extent? The fact that it is unnatural is not, in itself, an argument either way.

One of the methods used to in public discussions of going against nature is to argue in terms of categories. Holden and Vogel (2004) interviewed ethicists about the use of embryonic stem cells in research and treatment. The problem is that some people consider the use of these cells to be killing innocent human life, a category of acts that is considered wrong. (I shall discuss some answers to this claim in section 4.3.2.) Holden and Vogel describe their reactions to technical "fixes" that might get around this problem:

- In response to the idea of genetically modifying the embryo with a "knockout gene" so that it cannot form an organized embryo, Richard Doerflinger of the National Council of Catholic Bishops in Washington, D.C., argued, "If the knockout gene allows for several days of relatively normal development, then it would not solve the problem. A short-lived embryo is still an embryo."

- In response to the idea of using a parthenote, an embryo created from an unfertilized egg, Doerflinger said, "If [parthenotes] are organized enough to make a blastocyst, my concerns would still be there. The jury is out on what exactly a parthenote is, but I don't think it's been shown that it isn't an embryo."

- To the idea of using stem cells from nonviable embryos, Tadeusz Pacholczyk of the National Catholic Bioethics Center in Philadelphia, Pennsylvania, responded, "I'm not convinced that an arrested embryo is the same as a dead embryo, given the ability of single cells from early embryos to form entire organisms."

- Against the idea of growing stem cells from single cells that have been detached from embryos without damaging the embryos, Peter Braude, a stem cell researcher at Guy's, King's and St. Thomas' School of Medicine in London, pointed out that such cells may still have "the potential to develop into a full embryo. So in some eyes, destroying it to make an [embryonic stem] cell line is akin to destroying a complete embryo."

The reasoning in all these cases involves attaching a moral injunction to a category (embryo, which implies "human being"), and then arguing

that, given the vague boundaries of the category, we should avoid unnatural procedures that might arguably fall into that category. The critics
do not discuss what property of the category leads to the prohibition on
killing, and whether that property applies to the cases at hand.

Although all these arguments may be independently derived, it is
possible that some of them are the result of "myside bias" (Baron 1998).
Once having arrived at a position, people look for additional reasons to
support it (and fail to look quite so hard for reasons on the other side).
Manipulation of category boundaries is a way to find support.

4.2 Deficits and drugs

Learning disabilities and related disorders are worthy of separate discussion. Historically, learning disabilities were thought of as discrete syn-
dromes, probably with some biological cause. And, indeed, some developmental disorders in children can be classified this way—such as Down
syndrome, various other forms of mental retardation, and, of course,
blindness and deafness. Reading disability was originally thought of
as a specific deficit in reading "despite normal intelligence."

With about 100 years now of study of mental abilities and their relation to each other, a few facts have been clearly established. One is
that mental abilities correlate with each other. Most children who are
good at reading will be good at math. They will also have faster reaction
times and better memories for nonsense syllables. Both real abilities and
abilities measured on tests correlate with each other.

A second fact is that these correlations are not perfect. Indeed, some,
while still positive, are quite low. Abilities tend to correlate more highly
when they are related. Reading ability correlates more highly with other
language abilities (vocabulary, ability to learn foreign languages, ability
to repeat correctly a long nonsense word such as an unfamiliar name,
and so on) than these language abilities correlate with spatial abilities
(for example, ability to do puzzles quickly, understand graphs, or remember how to get from one place to another).

The first fact leads us to expect that children who are good at many
things will be good at reading too. But the second fact insures that this
expectation will not always be confirmed. Thus, it is possible *for any abil-*

ity to find children who are good at just about everything except that ability. These facts seem to explain most cases of what are called learning disabilities. We notice discrepancies in some areas more than others when the areas in question are so crucial in our educational system, such as reading. (I myself was deficient in baseball, but that was not so crucial.)

The same general principles surely apply to general behaviors—such as ability to pay attention, to sit still, and to keep working at a task. The absence of these abilities in some children who are otherwise "smart" has led to new classifications, such as "hyperactivity" and "attention deficit disorder." But these are just names for particular patterns that have to exist, given the fact that abilities are imperfectly correlated. Although there may be some cases with specific biological causes, most children diagnosed with these disorders are just at one end of a continuum. The cut point on the continuum is arbitrary.

Two further changes have happened in the United States and to some extent elsewhere. One is that children with learning disabilities (including reading disability and attention deficit disorder) are being given special treatment. In the United States, this is the result of the 1990 passage of the Americans with Disabilities Act and Individuals with Disabilities Education Act (with major amendments in 1997), which included these deficits along with blindness and physical disability and specified that schools and workplaces attempt to accommodate people with any disability.[2] The result is that children diagnosed with learning disabilities get to take more time on tests and other school work, through college. In elementary school, they are often assigned to special, smaller classes. Despite the possible stigma attached to the diagnosis, many parents go to several psychologists, if necessary, to obtain the diagnosis for the children because of the special privileges that come with it that come with it.

A second change, in the case of attention deficit disorder (ADD), is the use of drug treatment with stimulants such as amphetamine and Ritalin (methylphenidate). Such stimulants improve attention and learning, and (unlike other stimulants such as coffee) have the effect of actually reducing excessive activity. They are also somewhat addictive.

---

[2]See `http://ada.gov`.

It was once thought that stimulants were a specific treatment for a disorder. Given the lack of any clear diagnostic criteria for ADD, some neurologists argued that the way to diagnose it was to try a stimulant, and, if the child improved, then the child had ADD. Now we know that stimulants, on the average, improve attention and reduce activity for all children, regardless of their diagnosis (Rapoport et al. 1978, 1980).

Educational researchers have a standard way of dealing with problems such as this, called aptitude-treatment interactions (Cronbach and Snow 1977). The approach is based on consequences and is thus fully consistent with a utilitarian or decision-analytic view. If children are to be treated differently according to some categorization, such as a diagnosis or a test, then we need to show that this differential treatment improves outcomes compared to the alternatives. The categorization is the "aptitude." We need to show that treatment X is better than treatment Y for those in the category, and that treatment Y is better than treatment X for those not in the category. If treatment X is at least as good as treatment Y for both categories, then we have no reason to use treatment Y at all. (We might want to take cost into account in deciding whether one treatment is better than another.)

But the use of extra time for learning disabilities and stimulant drugs for ADD do not meet these criteria. No research (to my knowledge) shows this. Extra time helps everyone do better on the test. It does not make the test more predictive for anyone, unless the test is badly designed. At least this hasn't been shown.

The kinds of aptitude-treatment interactions that have been discovered seem to have to do with general intelligence or learning ability. Fast learners learn more from a class that moves quickly than one that moves slowly, and slow learners do the opposite. This is a real interaction. It implies that educational "tracking" is sometimes beneficial. But tracking has been done long before the current increase in special classes and drugs.

So what are we to do? The problem is that the kind of special education given to learning disabled students—that is, small classes and special help—could probably help everyone, but it is too expensive to give to everyone. On the other hand, it is a matter of degree. The total amount of learning might be increased if the resources now devoted to special education were spread more evenly so that all students had access to some of them, instead of giving some students a great deal of access and most students none at all. Or, it may turn out that a convincing aptitude-treatment interaction will be found.

In the case of stimulant drugs, the problem is more difficult, because it is not clear that the drugs are beneficial in the long term, or that they are not beneficial. If they are beneficial in the long run, taking into account their addictive dangers and possible long-term side effects, then why shouldn't everyone have the opportunity to take them? If they are not beneficial, why give them to anyone?

We might consider a strategy of giving stimulants to the worst learners. However, the utility of (let us suppose) raising someone's IQ by 10 points may be just as great if the original IQ was 120 than if it was 80. (Normal is 100, and 80 is considered borderline retardation.) Thus, it is not clear that such a strategy is best.[3]

What does not seem relevant is the argument sometimes made that "there are other ways to solve the problem." For example, we could spend more money on education, or change our expectations about what children should do. These other ways might improve matters more if everyone took stimulants. (With reduced expectations, stimulated children might learn more on their own, freed from the tyranny of lesson plans and classroom organization.) The fact that there is something else to do is relevant only if the use of one method reduces the effectiveness of the other, or if the alternative is less costly and we cannot afford both.

4.3   Reproduction

A number of new technologies—and some not so new—involve reproduction. These include abortion, invitro fertilization (IVF), and cloning. I will use the common-language terms to discuss cloning. Reproductive cloning is the creation of embryos from a person's cells, with the intention of creating a new person who is genetically identical to the person who provided the cells. Therapeutic cloning is the creation of embryos, or just stem cells, which will then be used to provide tissue for transplan-

---

[3]If we want to reduce inequality, the easiest way to do that is to tax the rich and provide benefits to the poor. This works directly on outcomes. The effect of education is indirect at best.

tation into the person who provided the cells or someone else, or to do some sort of research.

Most people find the idea of cloning to be upsetting. In my research (for example, Baron and Ritov 2005), I have found that many people say that reproductive cloning should never be done or allowed, no matter what the benefits. They are not willing to trade off their opposition to cloning with anything else, and they say that the issue arouses strong emotions—such as anger. I have not found any issue that arouses more emotion or stronger absolute values than reproductive cloning. Those who believe that the strength of our emotion and of our commitment is sufficient to define what we ought to do can stop here.

Abortion has been a subject of hot debate for many decades, but opinion about it is nowhere near so uniform as that about cloning. Many of the arguments are similar, however. Those who oppose abortion generally seem to treat their opposition as a protected value, and it arouses strong emotion, like cloning. Those who favor the right to abortion, in my research at least, seem not to have such strong views. (Many people oppose abortion and oppose banning it. Others regard it as an unfortunate necessity that is sometimes for the best.)

Therapeutic cloning is also controversial, in part because its potential benefits include the curing of disease, which is assumed to be a legitimate reason to go against nature (in contrast to improvement beyond the natural). It is still often opposed by those who oppose abortion because it involves the killing of embryos, just as abortion does.

4.3.1   Biases in judgment: the double effect

Some of the objections to reproductive technologies seem internally inconsistent. For example, one objection to therapeutic cloning is that it throws away embryos. Yet, the destruction of embryos after fertilization is a side effect of normal reproduction; more embryos are fertilized than develop into viable fetuses. People who do not want to destroy embryos should avoid unprotected sex. Destruction of embryos is also a by-product of IVF.

Can the critics of cloning distinguish it from normal reproduction or IVF? One distinction is that normal reproduction is natural. This appeal to nature would make both IVF and cloning immoral.

Another way to make the distinction is to distinguish intended side effects vs. unintended side effects, or direct harm vs. indirect harm. The basic idea goes back to Aquinas's argument that killing in self-defense is not immoral (1947, 2 IIII, Q. 64, art. 7), which came to be known as the doctrine of the double effect:

> Nothing hinders one act from having two effects, only one of which is intended, while the other is beside the intention. Now moral acts take their species according to what is intended, and not according to what is beside the intention, since this is accidental .... Accordingly the act of self defense may have two effects, one is the saving of one's life, and the other is the slaying of the aggressor. Therefore this act, since one's intention is to save one's own life, is not unlawful, seeing that it is natural to everything to keep itself in "being," as far as possible. And yet, though proceeding from a good intention, an act may be rendered unlawful, if it be out of proportion to the end.

Although Aquinas emphasized intention here, later writers found this concept difficult. Pascal and others noted, for example, that it could justify all sorts of immorality on the ground that intention was some good end served by the same behavior. For example, "Such is the way in which our fathers have contrived to permit those acts of violence to which men usually resort in vindication of their honor. They have no more to do than to turn off their intention from the desire of vengeance, which is criminal, and direct it to a desire to defend their honor, which, according to us, is quite warrantable" (Pascal 1941, p. 404). In a current example of the direction of intention, the Commonwealth of Pennsylvania does not permit the use of lethal drugs such as morphine for the purpose of euthanasia, but it does permit the use of the same drugs for the purpose of pain relief. It is thus legal for a physician to give morphine to a dying patient, knowing that the drug will hasten death by suppressing respiration, and desiring this result, so long as the "intent" is to relieve pain, even if the patient is comatose and therefore unlikely to feel pain. Once the intent of an act becomes separated from the act's foreseen and desired outcomes, intent can be anything at all. And, if it can justify one act, it can justify any act. The idea of intent thus cannot easily provide a clear distinction between, e.g., cloning and normal reproduction.

Later writers saw a less slippery distinction between direct harm and indirect harm. Quinn (1989), for example, says, "...a new and better formulation of the doctrine [of the double effect] ...distinguishes between agency in which harm comes to some victims, at least in part, from the agent's deliberately involving them in something in order to further his purpose precisely by way of their being so involved ...and harmful agency in which either nothing is in that way intended for the victims or what is so intended does not contribute to their harm."

The injunction against direct harm has also been attributed to Kant's second formulation of the Categorical Imperative: "Act so that you treat humanity, whether in your own person or in that of another, [1] always as an end and [2] never as a means only" (Kant, 1983). The negative injunction, "never as a means only," has been the source of much speculation. Because it contains the word "only," it is fully consistent with the view that those used as means must also be considered as part of the overall accounting. This view—that is, the utilitarian view—would make no distinction between direct harm and indirect harm. If Kant had accepted this utilitarian view, however, he would simply have said that everyone should count as an end, and the negative injunction would not have been needed. Perhaps Kant was indeed drawing on a more common intuition against the idea of using people as means at all: The use of people as means suggests harming them directly for the benefit of others.

Royzman and Baron (2002) found that people see the direct-indirect distinction as morally relevant. We presented subjects with hypothetical scenarios such as the following two (but without the "Direct" and "Indirect" labels):

> Scenario 1: Scientists planted a forest in order to preserve endangered species of trees and other plants. Most of the species in the forest are extinct everywhere else. The forest is now threatened by an infestation of insects. You are one of the scientists.
>
> If nothing is done, 10 species will become extinct.
>
> Direct option: You can spray the forest with a chemical that will destroy the plant species in which the insects make their

nests, thus killing the insects and saving the other plants.

Indirect option: You can spray the forest with a chemical that will destroy the insects. The same chemical will kill some of the plant species.

Scenario 2. You are a U.S. military base commander. A missile has just been mistakenly fired from your base at a commercial airliner. If nothing is done, 100 passengers will die.

Direct option: you can alter the course of another commercial airliner flying nearby so that it is placed in the path of the missile. The first airliner will be safe, but the missile will destroy the airliner whose course you change.

Indirect option: You can alter the course of the commercial airliner. The airliner will be safe, but the missile will destroy another commercial airliner flying right behind the first airliner.

In general, subjects preferred the indirect option; they thought it was more moral and less a cause of the bad aspect of the outcome. The same distinction might be relevant to therapeutic cloning. People may see the destruction of the embryo as a direct effect of the action rather than an indirect side effect. The embryos created in therapeutic cloning must in fact be destroyed in order to be used.

Of course, utilitarianism regards this distinction as irrelevant. What matters are the outcomes and their probabilities, not how they are achieved. From a utilitarian perspective, then, the preference for indirect harm is a bias in judgment.

4.3.2 Utility and reproduction

So how would a utilitarian decision analyst look at abortion and, more generally, reproduction? What are the utilities? In particular, how do we calculate the utilities of the unborn?

Utility is a relative scale. So the question is always, "compared to what?" There is no such thing as absolute utility—or zero utility—although we can adopt some state as a reference point. Utility is about comparing two outcomes.

So the answer is surprisingly easy when we are discussing what to do about a person who will be born anyway. If a pregnant woman plans to have her baby (i.e., not abort it), and if she is considering whether to take cocaine while she is pregnant, the relevant utility difference is that between the expected alternative lives of the child with and without prenatal cocaine exposure. We need statistical data for this, of course, and judgments of the utility difference between the two relevant expected lives. But it is not a special problem. The point is that neither option involves an abortion.

This point seems to be missed by some pro-choice activists who oppose any efforts to count drug use during pregnancy as a harm. In fact, it is a person who is harmed, not a fetus. Of course, it may be that criminal penalties are not the best way to deter such harm, but that is a separate question. It may also be that the law itself will be incapable of distinguishing between harm to a fetus and harm to the person that fetus will become, so that a legal recognition of the harm could set a precedent for a legal argument against abortion. So the pro-choice activists may be strategically correct, but only because others are irrational.

What if one of the options is abortion? Here we need to ask what is wrong with killing or preventing the existence of human life. Singer (1993) argues that there are two parts to the value of life. First, when we kill adult humans, we frustrate—to put it mildly—their goals, including the goal of experiencing and enjoying life. They cannot carry out any of their plans that depended on their existence. This part of utility depends on the existence of plans and values. It matters only if existing goals will be frustrated. Animals and infants do not have such plans and values, for they are the product of reflection.

The second part of the utility loss from killing is the loss of good experiences. Animals and infants can suffer this loss. Notice that this is simple experience. It does not depend on ongoing plans or memories (except insofar as people derive simple pleasure from plans and memories). Importantly, this type of utility does not depend on the being who has the experience. Because animals have only this type of utility (to a first approximation, anyway), they are "replaceable." We do no overall harm if we painlessly kill one animal and replace it with another.

Let us put aside the pain caused to the fetus by abortion itself. This is not an issue, we assume, when abortion is early enough. For late abortion, it is possible to prevent the pain with anesthesia, although I suspect it is rarely prevented. Putting this question aside, the main choice is between the existence or nonexistence of a new life.

Let us also put aside cases in which the abortion will protect the mother's health or life. If these cases are difficult at all, it is because of the difficulty of determining the fetus's utility.

From the perspective of simple pleasure, preventing a life is a harm. But it is also true that the life can be replaced. If the options under consideration do not change the total number of lives that will *ever* exist, then we do not need to consider the loss of pleasure. If, on the other hand, the number of lives expected to exist declines (perhaps by a fraction of a person, because of uncertainty) as a result of a decision to abort, then there is a loss, although there may also be offsetting gains resulting from a lower population in the world or within the family in question. It is unclear how close we are to the point where the world is so populated with humans that the additional pleasure that results from adding one more is balanced by the pain caused to others as a result of resource scarcity and pollution.[4]

As a matter of policy, the issue comes down to whether we want to increase the rate of population growth by discouraging abortion. Realistically, even if we want to increase the birth rate, we may do better to try to encourage more people to want children, on the ground that wanted children will come in to a better environment than children who were born only because of the force of law.

Let us turn now to the question of how to count the first kind of utility, the kind that arises from goals. I have argued that utility is goal achievement. (That view can encompass the pleasure view by assuming that pleasure can be expected to be a goal for everyone.) What is the utility of creating a goal and then letting it be partly achieved—as most goals are—if the alternative is not to create it at all?

We can evaluate utilities only in terms of the goals that affect the decision itself (Baron 1996a). Thus, the not-yet-existing goals do not count. What does count is the goals that others have for or against the creation

---

[4] And it surely matters where the additional child would be born. Many European countries have declining populations and are politically resistant to increased immigration from countries with too many young people. Given the resistance, the loss of a birth in these countries is surely a bad thing.

of new goals. In other words, the decision is up to us. The creation of new people—of the sort who have values and plans—has utility because we, who already exist, value it.

This conclusion concerns the creation of new people by any means, from the legal prohibition of abortion to the normal sexual reproduction of married couples. It is thus tempered by the same considerations concerning population that I just mentioned. As a matter of policy, if we decide that the birth rate is about right, and abortion is legal, then we have no reason to change anything. If we decide that the birth rate is too low, then outlawing abortion may not be the best way to increase it.

Now, there is a final issue here, and that is the moralistic utilities of those who oppose abortion—and those who support its legality. These are real utilities. People have utilities for the behavior of others. When others do something that goes against these values—such as have an abortion or prevent someone from having one—the holders of these values are hurt in a real way. Perhaps people should not have moralistic values, but they do.

To include such values in a decision analysis, we need to be careful to distinguish values from opinions about what to do, and, within values, to distinguish values for means from fundamental values. As I shall explain in sections 6.5.2 and 6.5.3, to elicit the relevant values (using money as a standard), we would need to ask questions such as, "Suppose that, in one day, 10 additional abortions are performed, beyond what is the daily normal amount, and you win some money in a lottery. How much money would you have to win in order to consider this combination of events to be neither better nor worse *for you*, on the whole, than if neither event happened?" Even this question does not eliminate means values. It is, of course, not a practical tool, since people would answer dishonestly if they knew how their answer would be used. Further refinement would be needed to make this kind of question practical.

Let us consider a practical case discussed somewhat in the literature on decision analysis (Deber and Goel 1990; Ganiats 1996), the utility of fetal testing. In the simplest case, a couple is determined to have a child, and the issue is which child it will have. The utility of fetal testing is roughly the difference in expected utility between the child that will be born with or without testing, minus the cost of testing C. Suppose the test is for Down syndrome, and the probability of that is P. Then, assuming that the utility of no test is 0 and the test is perfect and does not cause miscarriages, then the utility of a test is $P \cdot (U - V - A) - C$, where U is the utility of a normal child, V is the utility of a child with Down syndrome, and A is the disutility of an abortion (expressed as a positive number). Each U and V is the sum of the utilities for the child and the parents, and for others. The utility of a Down child for those other than the parents is probably negative (compared to no child), while the utility of a normal child might be positive, depending on the population situation.

To estimate the utilities for the child, we would have to ask people to rate the utility of a life with Down syndrome on a scale in which 0 was no life at all and 100 was a normal life. We cannot ask about "the rest of your life." That is an unfair question, because changing to a life with Down syndrome would mean giving up one's current plans.

The disutility of abortion should include the moralistic utilities of those opposed to it, as well as the moralistic utilities of those who oppose bringing children into the world who then must rely on others for their care. (Right now, the former are surely more prevalent.)

Suppose we think that the couple will have (or might have) one less child if the current one is aborted. Here the formula becomes $P \cdot (X - V - A) - C$, where X is the utility of no child being born in this case. If a Down syndrome child is worse than no child, then $X - V$ may be high enough to justify testing. In a situation of limited population, X may even be as high as U, which would lead to the same result for the two formulas. Finally, suppose that the chance of having a child is Q. Then the formula becomes $P \cdot ([QU + (1 - Q)X] - V - A) - C$; we simply take the probability-weighted average of the two formulas.

The role of moralistic and other social utilities (utilities for others) depends on who is making the decision. The calculations so far assume that it is a true utilitarian who weighs everyone equally. But a particular couple might weigh their own interests more than they weigh others'. To the extent to which their decision conflicts with the overall utilitarian calculation, they are doing less good than they could. This is a common occurrence, and it is not necessarily "bad" in the sense that it should be punished. (If it should, then people should also be punished for failing to aid the world's poor in whatever way they can do so, within the constraint that the poor gain more utility than they lose from helping; see Singer 1993.)

4.3.3 Cloning

Reproductive cloning has some possible uses (President's Council on Bioethics 2002, ch. 5): producing biologically related children in those who cannot have them, avoiding genetic disease, obtaining rejection-proof transplants, replicating a "loved one" who is dying, and reproducing great talents. Let us put aside the question of risk, which I already discussed, and assume that cloning is someday safe. Arguments based on risk do not justify a permanent ban on reproductive cloning, and that is what the critics of cloning seek.

We can question the motives behind these reasons for cloning, but, as I argued earlier, such questioning does not bear on the decision to ban something unless a ban will discourage bad motives enough to justify it. The trouble is that essentially all of the motives that support such uses of cloning (good and bad) are widespread and involved in many other decisions. Thus, use of a ban on cloning to discourage any particular motives is likely to be "a drop in the bucket." If, for example, we want to discourage the self-love that leads parents to want children like themselves (assuming that it is bad), or to discourage the arrogance that leads people to challenge traditional constraints (assuming that it is bad), then we need to look at a lot more than cloning. Many of the arguments for a ban on cloning are based on its questionable motives.

The President's Council on Bioethics (2002, ch. 5) brings up several other arguments about cloning. One is that the risk issue will not go away, even when cloning is medically safe and sure. In particular, cloning can change the "relationships within the family and between the generations, for example, by turning 'mothers' into 'twin sisters' and 'grandparents' into 'parents,' and by having children asymmetrically linked biologically to only one parent." The council's "ethical" conclusion is, "Cloning-to-produce-children would also be an injustice to the cloned child—from the imposition of the chromosomes of someone else, to the intentional deprivation of biological parents, to all of the possible bodily and psychological harms that we have enumerated in this chapter. It is ultimately the claim that the cloned child would be seriously wronged—and not only harmed in body—that would justify government intervention." Yes, this is a risk, but any change in law or custom has similar risks. And these bad effects are surely not certainties. They might be quite minor. I'm sure that arguments like this were made (quite reasonably) against the laws that banned polygamy, where such laws exist.

Other arguments are essentially forms of the naturalistic fallacy, which, of course, parallels the risk argument just made. For example, the Council on Bioethics argues: "Procreation is not making but the outgrowth of doing." Note the "is" here. The parallel to the risk argument is that any change has risks. Any change can have unforeseen consequences. But changes can also have unforeseen benefits. To take one random example, the replacement of horses with automobiles was motivated largely by a desire for speed and convenience, but it had unforeseen effects of both kinds: urban sprawl, on the one hand, and a solution to the problem of accumulating horse manure, on the other. Of course, we should try to foresee the effects of our decisions, but to abjure change because we are confident that the unforeseen effects will be all bad simply goes against past experience. (Perhaps the bad effects are remembered better, but that could happen because bad events are more memorable than good ones.)

The possibility of unforeseen consequences is always a problem for decision analysis. In practice, decision analysis makes little attempt to correct its conclusions for the existence of such consequences. For example, I know of no studies of whether unforeseen consequences are generally good or bad, and data of that sort would certainly be useful if one type of consequence did predominate over the other. If we had such data, we could apply some overall correction. But any particular obscure consequence, such as those imagined by the President's Council, seems too unlikely to have much effect on any analysis. If the foreseen consequences were to be included in this way, then the analysis must make a systematic effort to find them all and elicit expert probabilities. I suspect that this would be wasted time, as this sort of scraping of the bottom of the barrel would have little effect on the conclusion.

4.4   Extending life

If we can extend life by slowing the natural aging process, should we do it? Surely, we are free to try to cure the diseases that predominate in old age, such as cancer and heart disease. Although a crude, hedonistic util-

itarian calculus might say that the totality of pleasure would be greater
if we let the suffering old die sooner so that we could replace them with
younger people more quickly, the utility of life for adult humans is (as
I argued in section 4.3.2) based on the values that people have for their
plans, projects, and ongoing connections with others.

We may be able to do more (Juengst et al. 2003; Miller 2002; Vaupel, Carey, and Christensen 2003). Is aging itself a disease to be cured?
Should we try to live forever? This is often considered an "ethical" question, rather than a simple calculation of what is best—of the sort we
would try to use to decide who should pay for prescription drugs, for
example. I think it is considered "ethical" because, if we simply let the
research proceed without worrying about the consequences, something
bad might happen, although it isn't clear what. Thus, people want to say
that we should not proceed so quickly in this area, and they do not want
to have to answer the question "Why not?" by pointing to some fairly
clear negative consequence, so they say it is "ethical."

4.4.1   Consequences of extending life

Perhaps a general problem is that, if we start extending life, and then discover some very bad consequence of doing so, it will be politically very
difficult to go back. Younger people will think it is terribly unfair to have
shorter lives than their parents. This political problem alone provides a
very clear reason to be careful. We do not need ethics, just a reasonable
aversion to huge and irreversible risks.

In the meantime, we have many ways to learn about the consequences
of life extension. Life has been getting longer, and it has been doing that
at different rates in different populations. The consequences should thus
be fairly easy to study in the way that demographers and economists
usually study things. It may even be possible to find "instrumental variables" that lengthen the life span relatively suddenly and in a way that
is not confounded with other factors, such as the introduction of clot-
busting drugs. We also need time and research to figure out what to do
with old people. What are the economic consequences of raising the retirement age, or not raising it, while people live longer and longer past
it?

4.4.2   Population vs. longevity

A more interesting question, perhaps, is how we compare the utility of having, say, 8 billion people who live to age 100 on the average with that of 9 billion who live to age 90. This question assumes that an effort to increase longevity could go hand in hand with an effort to reduce population.

We might try to answer this question by simply adding up the pleasurable experiences that come from existence. If we did that, and if we assumed that extending the life span did not change the average amount of pleasure per year (a reasonable assumption, I think, since extension of the life span would probably delay not only death but also the usual symptoms of old age), then we could simply multiply the number of people by their average age to get the total utility. The choice in the last paragraph would be a close one, but it would favor the second option. We might look at the economic effects, but, assuming that we raise the ages for various milestones—including retirement—in proportion to the life span, then it is difficult to imagine much difference in terms of productivity, for example. The benefits of mature wisdom might be assumed to be roughly offset by the lost benefits of youthful flexibility.

But, I have argued (in section 4.3.2) that the utility of creating new people by increasing the population cannot be determined by simply adding up experiences. Creating new people is, I argued, a matter of creating goals. Our utilities for the creation of goals are not constrained by the assumption that only experiences matter.

Following this argument, it would make sense, then, to try to elicit public values for population. In principle, we could ask people directly about the trade-off between longevity and population. Of course, we would have to ask the respondents to assume that the policies they evaluate apply to future generations, after their own death. This would remove the self-interested reason to choose longevity.

Suppose that population stabilizes below a sustainable level, so that it would be possible to increase longevity without any ill effects from increased population. (This could be true within a geographical region, if not in the world.) If we suppose that research finds no ill effects, then it is difficult to think of any utilitarian objection to increasing longevity, even quite far.

Perhaps the biggest worry is that someone discovers a complete and safe cure for aging all at once. Everyone will want it. Yet, unforeseen consequences could result. It would take a while to figure out how to adjust legal and economic arrangements. If the cure were phased in gradually, who would get it first? Perhaps these are questions worth addressing before it happens. For example, it might make sense to give it first to those who have not yet started to age—a policy I advocate with a little personal regret—because they would get the greatest benefit, and the noticeable effects would be delayed, allowing more time for planning.

4.4.3 Should we accept our fate?

To conclude this section, I would like to answer a reviewer argued that utilitarianism has hidden values. The reviewer said, "Baron assumes that saving and prolonging life is the most fundamental 'good' to be preserved via a utilitarian calculus." Bioethicists such as Daniel Callahan (2003) raise similar points by questioning the value of medical research in general, as opposed to other values, such as solidarity and community. Callahan specifically disputes the value of trying to extend life as such. Callahan provides a number of consequentialist arguments, such as the view that old people are bored anyway, and less productive than their replacements would be. But these are empirical questions. Earlier in this chapter, I saw no reason to think that longevity would be good or bad on the whole; either could be true, depending on the balance of benefits and costs.

As for boredom, or more generally, the acceptance of death, isn't that an individual matter? My grandmother died at 92 from risky cancer surgery. She said she took the risk willingly because she was ready for her long and full life to end, without suffering, if that should happen. My grandfather also died at 92, but he had no more interest in letting go of life than he would have had at 32. Each of us may think that, at the age of 92, we would, or should, be more appreciative. Can we predict so well, though, how we will feel at the time? Although it seems greedy to want to live much more than the "alloted" time, what is so bad about it?

Arguably, the idea that we should value life less as we age may be an instance of what Elster (1983) calls "adaptive preference formation" or "sour grapes." We change our goals to fit what we think is possible. Of course, the resulting goals are real, and utilitarians should respect them. But, on the other hand, what if such goals are based on false beliefs? As I have argued (Baron 1996a), we do not necessarily serve people's good by respecting false goals. If people knew that life extension were possible, their value for life might remain stronger in old age.

A utilitarian view must admit this possibility, but it must also admit the possibility that life extension does indeed have sufficient negative consequences so that it should not be a research priority. (Miller [2002] argues that it is not in fact a research priority, in part because so many policy makers agree with Callahan.) It is an empirical question. If I seem here to be overvaluing life relative to other goods, it is because of a personal, fallible judgment of how the empirical facts will turn out. It is not a consequence of utilitarianism itself.

4.5 Conclusion

To end on a more mundane note, the Associated Press reported on Dec. 4, 2003:

> Sacramento, California—Citing ethical concerns, state regulators Wednesday refused to allow sales of the first bioengineered household pet, a zebra fish that glows fluorescent. GloFish are expected to go on sale everywhere else next month.

> California is the only state with a ban on genetically engineered species, and the Fish and Game Commission said it would not exempt the zebra fish from the law even if escaped fish would not pose a threat to the state's waterways.

> "For me it's a question of values, it's not a question of science," said commissioner Sam Schuchat. "I think selling genetically modified fish as pets is wrong."

Where the wrongness comes from is, for Mr. Schuchat, not the consequences, although he might have some vague worries about them. It is the idea of tampering with nature. Yet humans have been tampering with nature since our species existed (Easterbook 1995). The great plains of the United States were once forests, and the "natural" forests of the east are mostly what has taken hold after the original ones were almost clear cut for wood. This is not to say that it is OK to wreck nature because we've been doing it all along. Rather, it is to say that what people take as a value for pristine nature is based to some extent on false beliefs.

I have argued in this chapter that we have an intuitive heuristic of judging what is good by what is natural. This is a useful heuristic, but it is overextended to the point of causing unnecessary harm in several domains: the development of new drugs, the limitation of some drugs to those with "diseases," limitations on reproduction, and possibly insufficient research on life extension. Each of these claims hinges on the facts of the case at hand. But the ubiquity of this intuitive principle makes me suspect that people will look harder for facts to support it than for facts on the other side.

Some bioethicists express what I take to be a kind of nostalgia, in which they doubt that "progress" is so great. They seem to long for the days when humans had less power against nature. Surely some progress is illusory: we invent suburbs, then build expressways to get to work, then invent amusements for the hours spent stuck in traffic on expressways, and cures for the diseases caused by the excess pollution, and on and on. But life, freedom from pain, and physical and mental capacity—that is, health—seem very close to fundamental values for almost everyone. It may be moralistic to try to prevent these values from expressing themselves in the marketplace and in the political arena.

Chapter 5

Death and the Value of Life

When I was on the Ethics Committee of the Hospital of the University of Pennsylvania (from about 1993 to 1997), we had monthly meetings, and the members of the committee were "on call" for consultations, which were usually reported at the next monthly meeting. Both the monthly meetings and the consultations were predominantly about dying patients. The typical consultation involved an elderly patient who was terminally ill, semiconscious, and suffering pain or discomfort. Generally, someone—either one of the hospital staff or one of the family members—would suggest either a "do not resuscitate" order or, if the patient was on some sort of life support, pulling the plug. Someone else, usually a family member (but once the attending physician) would then oppose the suggestion. The consultation was a guided negotiation between the two sides, in which everyone present had a say. (The combined skills of a mediator and a family psychotherapist might have been useful in the committee members, but they were not always present.) In the monthly meetings, we discussed general issues such as the pros and cons of withdrawal of tube feeding. The members of the committee frequently referred to "our view" as the view that decisions such as this had to be made, and that the preservation of life at all costs was not the single-minded goal of modern medicine. To the members of the committee, by and large, "ethics" meant deciding about life and death.

By what criteria should such decisions be made? More generally, what is the value of life? These issues will come up again in chapter

9; here, I shall deal with questions that pertain more to individual lives. (In chapter 9, I discuss the role of valuation in allocation of treatments.)

5.1   The value of life and health: QALYs

Medical decision analysis usually measures the value of interventions in quality-adjusted life years (QALYs). The idea is that the utility of health adds up over time. So we try to measure the utility of being in a given health state at a given time, and we add up these utilities over time (or integrate them, as the term is used in calculus).

Several methods are used to elicit judgments about these utilities. One of them, the time trade-off (TTO) is directly related to the theoretical assumption behind the QALY idea. We ask, "How many future years in good health, followed by death, is just as good as 20 years with angina, followed by death?" The description of the angina can be quite detailed, or the judge could be a patient evaluating his own condition. Suppose the answer is 15 years. Then we conclude that the utility of angina is .75 on a scale where 0 is death and 1.00 is good health. This is because 15 years in good health is 15 QALYs, and, therefore, 20 years with angina must be 15 QALYs, and .75 multiplied by 20 is 15.

Other methods may ask just about the conditions without bringing time into the judgment question. For example, the simplest, the rating method, is just to ask, "On a scale where 100 is good health and 0 is immediate death, where would you put angina?" (See Baron 2000, ch. 13, for discussion of the main methods and their difficulties.)

5.1.1   Advantages of QALYs

The QALY method approach has several advantages, especially for the analysis of health policy. It allows the comparison of benefits of medical interventions on a common scale. It is thus the basis of most cost-effectiveness analysis in health. We can compare the QALYs per dollar of medical interventions. The common view is that interventions that cost more than $100,000 per year are questionable, although surely this figure is increasing over time. Most of the things covered by health insurance are more cost-effective than this. The ability to compare interventions in cost-effectiveness is a major tool for efficient allocation: if we reduce funding for interventions that are very costly and increase funding for those that are more cost-effective, we can improve health and/or reduce spending on it (as discussed in chapter 9).

Note also that the same approach applies to lifesaving. Saving a life is, from the point of view of cost-effectiveness, simply a matter of increasing the number of QALYs. If a QALY is worth $100,000, then saving the life of a 30-year-old with a future life expectancy of an additional 50 years in good health is worth $5,000,000, which is in the right ballpark with the numbers that many experts think should be the standard figure for the monetary value of saving the lives of random people (in rich countries). Of course, the QALY idea implies that interventions that save the lives of the very old are not as worthwhile. Although some people intuitively object, claiming that "a life is a life," others feel that the distinction is fair, since older people have already had their "fair share" of life, and the young should therefore have priority.

5.1.2 Whose values?

Several studies have asked whether patients who are actually experiencing some condition might evaluate it differently from those who simply imagine it. Some studies find that those with a condition assign it a higher utility (i.e., closer to normal health) than those without it (see Ubel, Loewenstein, and Jepson 2003, for a recent review), although other studies find a reversed effect for some conditions (Baron et al. 2003). Whose values are correct? Whose values should be used in cost-effectiveness analysis? The answer surely depends on the source of this discrepancy.

One possibility is that nonpatients may fail to think of the possibilities for adapting to handicaps. There are several sources of adaptation. One is the use of special devices, such as text-to-speech computer programs for the blind. People may also learn how to get around their handicaps. Failure to think of these things is simply an error that must be corrected if the values of nonpatients are to be used.

On the other side, some adaptation may happen because people change their goals to adapt to what they can do (Elster 1983). People who become blind can lose their interest in the visual arts and in the beauty of nature, thus being less frustrated by their handicap. Should we take this into account in evaluating the disutility of blindness?

It is beside the point whether this change of goals is rational for the patients themselves. Surely, one property of a goal that we might consider when deciding whether to bring it into existence or increase its strength (or the reverse) is whether it can be achieved. If we make decisions that favor creation of goals that are achievable over goals that are not, we can increase total utility. Changing goals can also be irrational. People sometimes "give up too soon." They convince themselves that something is unachievable and stop wanting it, when, in fact, they could achieve it (Elster 1983). For example, with effort, people with severe handicaps can work.

When we decide how much money to spend on the prevention of blindness, for example, it may not be correct to consider the fact that blind people will change their goals to adapt to their handicap. We may do better to honor the goals of the people who have not yet become blind, before adaptation. Arguably, these are the people who matter. We should, however, make sure that, when they evaluate blindness, they consider the pressure to change their goals as part of what blindness means. This consideration can make blindness seem less bad, because of the adaptation of goals, but worse because of the need to change the goals. This need may itself be undesired.

If the question is cure rather than prevention, then the people affected are those with the condition. If their goals are rationally chosen, then we should honor them. We may find ourselves placing a higher value on the prevention of a condition than on its cure, because those with the condition have rationally adapted to it. This need not be as crazy as it sounds. If the adaptation is irrational—a "sour grapes" effect—then we should ignore it and treat both groups, those who do not have the condition yet and those who have it, equally.

The general point is that we should try to consider fundamental goals or values, not those that result from false beliefs about what happens or what is possible. Many of these false beliefs result from self-deception.

5.1.3 Problems with QALYs

Although the QALY idea is a simple and straightforward application of the utilitarian point of view, it has problems even from that perspective. One is that QALYs count everyone as equal. This is intuitively fair and politically correct, but surely not true in terms of utilities. For one thing, the equality assumption ignores the value that people have for other people's lives. The death of a person embedded in a family is surely worse than the death of an otherwise equivalent person who is a complete loner. To conclude otherwise is to say that human attachments count for nothing. To take an extreme case, the utility of the lives of infants and young children is surely increased by the attachments that their parents have to them (as discussed in section 4.3.2).

The main argument against considering such factors in the analysis of health-care decisions is that the health system is not set up to evaluate the value of people to others. Indeed, it isn't just family ties that matter but also productivity and importance in a social system. Once we start evaluating the value of individual lives, it is difficult to figure out where to stop. From a practical point of view, it seems reasonable not to burden the health system with such calculation and limit setting. It is also a strong intuition. When Governor Robert Casey of Pennsylvania had a heart-lung transplant, many were suspicious that he had jumped ahead in the queue because he was governor. It may not have been so bad if that had happened, but apparently it didn't.

A related issue is the value of lives of disabled people. A typical finding is that people place some utility on preventing or curing serious disabilities such as paraplegia or blindness, but they also think that saving the lives of blind people or people in wheelchairs is just as important as saving the lives of people without a disability. The trouble is that the numbers do not add up (Ubel, Richardson, and Pinto Prades 1999). If, for example, preventing blindness is worth 20 on a 0–100 scale, where 0 is death and 100 is normal health without disability, and preventing a death (of anyone, blind or not) is worth 100, then preventing someone from dying and from being blind is worth 120, which is more than preventing a sighted person's death, even though the ultimate consequences are the same—one sighted person alive who would otherwise be dead.

Such intuitions may arise by thinking about changes rather than states. Learning that you were saved from death and blindness might be truly more gratifying than learning that you were saved from death alone. It is also possible that the intuitions result from underestimation of the value of life as a blind person: 80 may be much too low. But it is likely that the basic intuition here is that "we just don't make judgments about the relative value of people's lives." Thus, we switch between two modes of thinking. In one, we value blindness as a disability; in the other, we value blind people's lives as lives (as suggested by the results of Oliver 2004). The apparent contradiction is a consequence of adopting a principle of valuing all lives equally. Again, from a strictly utilitarian point of view, this is an error. The lives of blind people are statistically worse than the lives of others, at least a little. So, on the average, saving blind people does less good. But we want to avoid the disputes involved in making this kind of judgment, so we refuse to make it.

A second problem with the idea of QALYs, much less serious, is that they ignore the utility of lives as wholes. If humans were like other animals, then most of the things that we value would concern experiences. Experiences do add up over time. (We should also count the memories of experiences as experiences in their own right, in order to account for the fact that memories are not simple additive functions of experiences over time; see Kahneman et al. 1993.) But, unlike the case of the value of life for others, it is difficult to think of cases in which the QALY idea is a terrible approximation to the value of health and life.

A third problem with QALYs is the meaning of death, when we say that 0 represents death on the utility scale. The use of death could present practical problems for subjects who make judgments. Good health and angina are states, and we can imagine living in these states. But death is not a state. We do not imagine living in a state of death.[1] Thus, when we

---

[1] Of course, religious people who believe in life after death can imagine a "state of death," and this may lead such people to value their lives on earth less, if they think that the state of death will be a good one. However, entering the state of death, in most religious views, means largely or completely giving up one's earthly plans and projects, and giving up those projects is a lot of what is bad about death. Life after death would be similar in value to reincarnation, except that memories of life on earth would remain. Reincarnation itself should be of no value: It is no better for *me* if I die and am reincarnated as a frog, who remembers nothing of my life, than if I simply die. Even if that frog turns out to be a prince.

answer questions about health states, most of us are really comparing three prospects: living some number of years in good health; living the same number of years with some disorder; and death, with all that entails, including the failure to carry through plans for the future. We think about the overall desirability of the prospects rather than the experiences that we have in them.

The fact that death is a transition, not a state, in itself is not such a problem, but it becomes a larger problem if we equate this kind of transition from life to death with the state of nonexistence that comes about as a result of not being born (section 4.3.2). This equation is a mistake, if only because the transition from life to death involves giving up plans. We must be careful to avoid this equation, although, in fact, it is not a problem in all examples of cost-utility analysis I have seen, all of which involve decisions about living people.

The QALY approach has direct implications for decisions made about life-sustaining treatment for very sick people. It implies that many such treatments are likely to be wasteful, in the sense that they are much less cost effective than many things that could be done—but are not done— for healthier people. If people understood this implication, they may prefer insurance policies that limit expenditures at the end of life, while perhaps increasing the availability of more cost-effective measures, such as some of the more effective but expensive methods of cancer screening (such as colonoscopies every few years for those over 50).

5.2   Advance directives

People can make decisions about end-of-life care through advance directives, which usually specify what they want done for themselves in the way of treatment (living wills), and who is to be consulted about decisions or empowered to make decisions (power of attorney). One question is whether people are able to make such judgments, especially those about medical treatment. Current practices do not make such judgments easy for them.

5.2.1   Meaningful survival

Many forms used for living wills ask patients to specify which treatments they would want in order to prolong their lives. It is not clear that patients' expressed desires for these treatments reflect their underlying values. Patients may misunderstand the nature of each treatment. A focus on treatments, although helpful in making decisions, may not help the patient to reflect on important values.

An alternative approach is to ask each patient what constitutes meaningful survival for him. Patients can be asked how much (or whether) they would desire to live under various conditions. Patients cannot be expected to anticipate all the possibilities here, so they ought to be provided with a framework. It may turn out that the framework could be very simple. For example, a single dimension might suffice, corresponding to the overall degree of impairment: Some patients may desire aggressive treatment, even when they are highly impaired, and other patients may desire relatively little treatment. Or, it may turn out that two dimensions characterize most people's concerns, such as physical and mental capability. Of course, any form for patients should allow patients to express idiosyncratic preferences. But patients would probably find it helpful to be reminded of the major dimensions that most people care about.

To discover the dimensions, researchers could first assemble a set of items concerned with meaningful survival by searching the literature and by asking people to think of situations in which they would (and would not) want to be kept alive. It may even turn out that items from existing scales can be used for this purpose, such as the EuroQoL.[2] Then, a new sample of subjects would rate the importance of each item for meaningful survival. Application of factor analysis to the answers may discover a small number of dimensions. That is, roughly, some groups of items may correlate with each other so highly that only one or two items from the group may be needed to get most of the information about where each person stands on the items in the group. A questionnaire based on this analysis could be checked against specific vignettes, each including the current condition of the patient, a treatment that is being

---

[2]http://www.euroqol.org

considered, and the range of possible outcomes (when more than one outcome is possible).

5.3   Euthanasia and assisted suicide

Questions about life-sustaining treatment shade into questions about passive and active euthanasia and assisted suicide. In most legal jurisdictions, active killing is illegal but passive "letting die," by omission, is legal. Note that "pulling the plug" is not counted as an action, from a legal point of view. Withdrawal of treatment is considered an omission and is therefore legal. Withdrawal of hydration and feeding is borderline but is still mostly legal. In sum, it is legal not to undertake activities that cause life to be sustained, but it is illegal to undertake activities that cause death.

An interesting exception concerns medication for pain relief. In some jurisdictions (such as Pennsylvania), it is legal to provide morphine for pain relief, knowing that it will hasten death through suppression of respiration, but also knowing that the morphine would not be prescribed if it did not have this suppressive effect, so long as the "purpose" is to relieve pain. This is a classic example of the doctrine of the double effect at work (section 4.3.1). Interestingly, it seems that this is possible even for patients who are in a coma, hence, presumably, cannot feel pain. The intended purpose of relieving pain does not need to pass a rationality test. The law here still follows the general pattern of classifying activities by their purposes, but morphine in this case has a dual purpose, and the law allows the more "benign" one to count.

From a utilitarian perspective, it is the consequences that matter. If the only consequence is death without suffering, and this is considered to be good, then it does not matter how the outcome is achieved. In many cases, active euthanasia is preferable to waiting for death from natural causes, as the latter may involve greater suffering, beyond the point at which the patient would rather die than suffer. The prohibition of active euthanasia and assisted suicide seems to be a simple example of omission bias at work (sections 3.1.2 and 9.1.1).

5.3.1 Errors

It may turn out, as a matter of fact, that legalization of active euthanasia would lead to more errors in which people were mistakenly killed, or the opposite error in which people suffer too much.

Active euthanasia (including assisted suicide) may be done at any time, without waiting for a condition to become severe. Many actual cases of assisted suicide are people who are beginning a long decline from a degenerative disease. The cost of errors in such cases could be high. A person could be helped to die, and then a cure for her disease could be found. Something like this might have happened with some AIDS patients who missed out on antiretroviral drugs that could have allowed them to return to an almost-normal life. If a person with decades to live makes a mistake, much more is lost than if a person is allowed to die who is likely to die within weeks in any case.

The opposite error could also occur: a person could suffer greatly out of some vain hope that a cure would be found.

A decision analysis of this situation should consider the probability of errors of each type, the disutility of each error relative to the optimal decision, and the cost of decision making itself. Note that many errors will have little loss, because the situation is really close to a toss-up (as later discussed in section 6.2). These errors will be the most likely. Large errors, with a great loss in utility, will be less likely. So what is really needed is a function that tells us how probability of error depends on disutility for the two types of errors and, within each error, for different levels of disutility. We would compute the expected disutility of each error type by multiplying the probabilities by the respective disutilities and adding them up.

The cost of decision making would include various provisions for reducing errors, such as requiring more thorough review of decisions that are more likely to lead to large errors. This is essentially what is done in the Netherlands and the state of Oregon. The increased review may take the form of mandatory waiting periods for assisted suicide, or a requirement that disinterested doctors review the case and give their permission.

At this point, it simply is not clear where the chips will fall. If I am correct that much of the opposition to euthanasia and assisted suicide comes from omission bias, then it seems likely that some rule more liberal than the current distinction based on action versus omission will be superior, perhaps something like what is being done in the Netherlands or Oregon. Data from these experiments will help others decide. Note that these experiments cannot be expected to be free of mistakes. We must, however, take into account the fact that a total ban on active euthanasia also causes mistakes that lead to intense suffering, and we must balance one sort of mistake against another. The measurement of QALYs will give us an approximate way to do that, and, given that many choices will be toss-ups, that is probably sufficient.

5.3.2   Social pressure and altruism

Another issue often raised in discussions of assisted suicide or euthanasia is that, if these practices become common, people will feel more compelled to die for the benefit of others. They will face social pressure, the pressure to conform and to do what others expect them to do. In particular, people will forgo their current right to have a lot of money spent on postponing their deaths for a short time, or on maintaining life in the face of suffering that makes life barely worth living. Putting this another way, current law and ethical practice do not require people to consider the effects of their end-of-life decisions on others.

Sometimes, we actively discourage excessive altruism. Donation of organs from living donors is rarely done when the risk to the donor is moderately high, even when the donors are willing and fully informed about the risks.

Note first that this issue already exists, given the legality of passive euthanasia. People who complete living wills are often aware of the large amounts of money that can be spent at the end of their lives. They may think of themselves as selfish to demand such expenditures. Other people are willing to forgo treatment because they do not want to be a burden on their families in terms of their need for time and care, even if their medical expenses are covered. A liberalization of the laws concerning death would increase the pressure but not create it.

We need to distinguish the issue of pressure to be altruistic from a related issue, which is the possible rationing of health care (chapter 9). When expensive end-of-life care is not covered by insurance and the patient cannot pay for it, then the issue of altruism just does not come up. People die sooner as a result of not being able to pay for the treatment themselves and not having it covered. This is a policy decision that causes some people to die sooner, possibly against their will, so that others can have some benefit, possibly even a longer life. What is at issue here is treatments that are covered by insurance and hence optional. It may turn out, however, that more stringent criteria for insurance coverage would reduce the pressure to be altruistic (just as legal liberalization might increase it). In particular, people would worry less about taking more than their fair share if they felt that their share was strictly limited.

What, then, is the disutility of pressure to be altruistic? We are, again, not talking about forcing people to forgo their preferred option in favor of an option with less utility. Rather, the issue is the loss that results when people voluntarily choose an option that helps others and hurts themselves, but those same people would not do so if they did not feel social pressure.

One possible argument is that social pressure is just what happens when consequences for others come to a person's attention. The person may have altruistic fundamental values but not realize how relevant these values are to the case at hand. If the social pressure is part of a complete set of information, then all it does is help people to realize their fundamental values in their decisions. Thus, it is not harmful. What is harmful is the withholding of *any* information that might bear on the decision, including information on the other side—such as the possibility of a more complete recovery from illness than was thought possible at first, or the possibility of a research breakthrough.

Also harmful is the provision of false or misleading information. If the family exaggerates the difficulties they would have caring for their disabled uncle, he could be tricked into a decision to forgo treatment. Perhaps those who worry about social pressure feel that it is so difficult to police such trickery that it would be best to reduce the opportunity for it by not liberalizing the laws about death—that is, by reducing choice. So the idea is to reduce choice lest people be tricked into making bad choices. Any reduction in choice, of course, eliminates the benefits that can come from choice—namely, the tailoring of decisions to individual utilities. These decisions may differ from the option provided when choice is absent.

In principle, we could try to estimate the probability and utility loss from trickery, and the probability and utility loss from limiting choice. These would be the relevant factors in a decision analysis. The fact that they are difficult to estimate does not imply that any other approach is going to yield a better decision than reliance on fallible estimates.

Choice limitation might maximize utility in some situations. But it seems likely to me that some fundamental bias is involved in the fear of social pressure, rather than a correct intuition that choice reduces utility. Perhaps the bias is in the idea that people have a right to be selfish, especially when that selfishness can be expressed as an omission. A social expectation of being willing to die has the effect of turning unwillingness into an act, hence it becomes a positive expression of selfishness.

5.4 Organ donation and the definition of death

An apparent example of selfishness by omission is the failure to donate organs. Organ donation is related to death, however. Some of the fears that people have about donating organs are that they will be allowed to die sooner—perhaps even when they could still recover their health—because the hospital staff was overeager to get their organs in order to help someone else.

Another issue is that, even when death is certain, the definition of death that must be used is so stringent that organ donation is impossible, or rendered less effective. Some religious groups hold that death requires the cessation of the heart; this is usually too late for healthy organ procurement. Yet, "brain death" is surely a matter of degree, and sometimes it is more difficult to determine, although there are standard tests that can be used to make a somewhat arbitrary decision quickly.

One of the virtues of decision analysis in general is that it does not need to deny the possibility of error. Surely, any definition of death that allows transplantation of the most vital organs is going to lead to some errors. A liberal definition of death, however, seems likely to lead to very few such errors. And when they happen, their disutility would probably be very low. Most of them would lead to a slight shortening of a life that would soon end anyway, possibly with great benefit to someone else.

5.5   Conclusion

Medical decision analysis usually values life as if it were a container, without trying to assign value to what it contains. The relevant unit is a life year adjusted for its quality, a QALY. Lives in "good health" are valued equally, even though "good health" may include a severe handicap. Medical decision analysis, as an institution, limits its role in this way in order to stay within its expertise. The task is to measure health for each person on a common scale, not to function as a utilitarian government. The important achievement is the common scale. This allows decision makers to compare one intervention to another. The idea that goodness can be compared across different means of achieving goodness is the great insight of utility theory in general, and it is a useful insight, even though it does not solve every problem.

Many of the problems of utility measurement may result from this limitation of its role. For example, it can tell us that saving a person's life while simultaneously curing his chronic handicap, thereby restoring a person to health without the handicap, can have more utility than saving the life of a person without the handicap. This apparent inconsistency may result in part from the insistence that the lives of the two people had equal utility at the outset.

Utilities are difficult to measure, and they are thus measured with considerable error. This error may not matter, because it may not affect any decision. If it matters, often the decision is a close one, so making the wrong choice will have little expected cost, when compared to the correct choice. Moreover, decision analysis may reveal the true source of difficulty.

This chapter has illustrated some of the sources of difficulty and made some suggestions about how to deal with them. Some sources, such as the distinction between acts and omissions, are more apparent than real. Other sources can be handled by an analysis of error in the analysis itself. In other cases, such as the problem of altruism, I think that a decision-analytic approach can help us understand the true conflicting issues.

Chapter 6

Coercion and Consent

The idea of informed consent is a major contribution of modern bioethics. If the victims of Nazi experiments and of the Tuskegee study had been fully informed and free to participate or not, they would not have suffered. On the other side, it is remotely possible that Jesse Gelsinger would not have died (see chapter 1) if the parents of infants born with his condition had been deemed capable of consenting. The effort to protect autonomy even from the pressures of emotion can result in what might be interpreted as excessive paternalism.

For most bioethicists, informed consent grows out of a principle of autonomy and "respect for persons." Yet, this principle is not absolute even for those who honor it. Utilitarian decision analysis can help us to make trade-offs with other principles. It can also help us to understand the benefits of autonomy itself.

6.1 The value of choice

The main benefit of autonomy is that what is best for each of us depends on our individual values (utilities). Each of us generally knows more about our own values than others know about them. Thus, even if others tried to make the best decision for us, they would usually not do as well as we would do by ourselves at maximizing our own utility.

The situation is worse still when others try to do something other than maximize utility, for example, when they try to impose their moralistic values on us (section 3.1.4). Autonomy is a good defense against having values imposed on us by others.

Autonomy is less important when choices do not depend on individual values. This can happen when the relevant outcomes can be described in terms of a single number that is the same for everyone, such as an amount of money or the probability of death. In general, we can assume that everyone prefers more money, and a lower probability of death. Such decisions do not arise very often. An apparent advantage of cost-benefit analysis is that it converts all values to money, thus allowing this sort of one-dimensional reasoning, but the conversion to money makes assumptions about individual values that may not hold. In particular, a given improvement in health need not have the same monetary value to everyone.

Autonomy has additional values of a psychological sort. Although people dislike making decisions that involve allocation of goods to others (Beattie et al. 1994), they generally prefer to choose between options A and B than to simply get the better of the two options, they regard the choice as having more utility than the best option, and they value the best option more when it is chosen than when it is not (Beattie et al. 1994; Bown, Read, and Summers 2003; Szrek 2005). To some extent, these results may be illusory. For example, people know that choice usually leads to better outcomes for themselves than lack of choice, so they may assume that this is true in every case, even when the option they get is the same whether they choose it or not. This would be an example of an overapplication of a heuristic. Yet, the actual utility of the chosen option, for achievement of their goals, may be the same whether they choose it or not. Yet, the illusion is not the whole story. If people are happier with choice, then the happiness itself has utility for them.

Excessive choice has harmful consequences (Iyengar and Lepper 2000, 2002; Schwartz et al. 2002). When people have too many choices, they are more likely to accept the default, even when that is the status quo and when many options are superior to it, and they are often less satisfied with the option that they get. Note that these negative effects of choice have not been found for small sets of options, such as two options vs. one option. The results seem to depend on the difficulty of the choice itself, and the possibility of regret from missing some option that might have been better. The problem of excessive choice is most relevant for consumer decisions, when, even in a grocery store, consumers in rich countries are faced with a bewildering array of options in every aisle.

In medical decisions, the problem can arise in such cases as fetal testing, when we increasingly find the same sort of bewildering array of options. It may be that the use of formal decision analysis can make decisions easier, hence less aversive and less likely to induce regret.

6.2   The flat maximum

An important principle from decision analysis is the "flat maximum" (von Winterfeldt and Edwards 1986, section 11.4). Suppose we have several options, such as having one child, having two, having three, or having four. Or the options could be academic courses, vacations, or medical treatments. Suppose we carry out a decision analysis to compute the utility of all the options. Under fairly general conditions, the two options with the highest utility will be fairly close.

Why is this? Von Winterfeldt and Edwards give three general reasons. First, when you select the best options in a decision analysis, you have already eliminated options that are dominated. Option A is said to dominate option B if A is better than B in some way and worse than B in no way. Thus no trade-off is involved in choosing A over B.

Figure 6.1 shows how this might work with several options that vary in price and quality, with higher utility going to the right on price (hence low prices are to the right) and upward on quality. Options A, B, and C dominate all the others. For example, the price of option C is just as low as the price of option g, yet the quality of C is higher. So the analysis of the decision among these options would focus on A, B, and C. The choice depends on the trade-off between price and quality—that is, the relative utility of a given change in price vs. a given change in quality. If the utility of a change in price is high enough, then option C will be chosen, but B will not be far behind. Similarly, if quality matters more, A will be chosen, but B will not be far behind. And, if B is the best, either A or C will be fairly close.

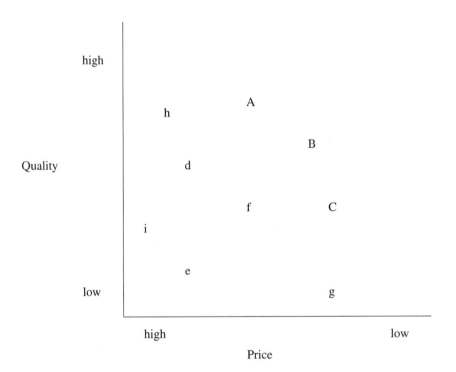

Figure 6.1: Illustration of how dominance leads to a flat maximum

The second reason for the flat maximum is that most decisions that are worth thinking about are close calls. We do many things in life without thinking, and, in most cases, the best thing to do is totally obvious. When a deer runs in front of your car, you step on the brakes. But the decisions discussed in this book are presumably not of this type. Presumably they are worth discussing. In these cases, the very closeness that makes them worth discussing also implies that one option is typically not much better than another. So there is little loss from choosing the second best option. (On the other hand, as von Winterfeldt and Edwards point out, analysis sometimes reveals that options once thought to be close are not close at all.)

The third reason for the flat maximum is that most decision analysis involves weighted averages. We weigh utilities by probabilities in expected-utility analysis, and we weigh attribute utilities by attribute weights in multiattribute analysis. We often feel uneasy about the probabilities or the attribute weights. However, adjustment of these rarely changes the conclusion. And when the conclusion is changed by such adjustment, the difference between the new best option and the old best option is small. In other words, if a decision analysis is carried out with error, so that the wrong option is chosen, this is because the options were close to begin with, and the utility loss from choosing the wrong option is small.

This point is intuitively difficult for some people. Usually, we think that close decisions are worth a great deal of thought. That is true if our goal is to be sure that we have chosen the best option. However, if our goal is to maximize utility, we need to trade off the utility loss from further thinking with the utility gain from whatever improvement can result from that thinking. And the improvement is typically small, because the very thing that makes the decision seem "difficult" is that the options are truly close. Thus, while it is true that choosing which college to go to will affect the future course of a student's life in major ways, the nature of these effects is difficult to foresee, and most students will do well by narrowing the choice to the two best options and flipping a coin (and, of course, flipping it again if it comes out the wrong way).

We tend to take a similar attitude toward autonomy. We think that an autonomous decision is the one that someone would make totally without influence from others. Yet, if the influence is weak and still effective, the difference in utility between the decision finally made and the one that would have been made without the influence is probably small. And, if the influence serves some purpose, some other sort of utility may increase as a result.

An example is the use of persuasive communications to "sell" the idea of birth control to people in countries with very high rates of population growth (Baron 1998, ch. 8). For example, some governments and nongovernmental organizations have carried out advertising campaigns to encourage smaller families. One organization, Population Communication International (http://www.population.org) even helps to produce radio and TV soap operas that deal with family issues in a way that encourages smaller families. Some people regard these persuasive efforts as interference with the autonomous right of families to decide for themselves how many children to have.

From a utilitarian perspective, autonomous decision making is important in part because it results in more good. That happens because individuals know more about their own good than others do, on the average. One of the advantages of a capitalist economy, with much choice of goods, is that people can choose what maximizes their utility, regardless of what others choose. Some people like Microsoft Windows because it allows easy interaction with other Windows users (and it has good games). Other people like Linux because it is more easily customized and more versatile. If the latter were forced to use Windows, they would suffer, and vice versa.

A second utilitarian advantage of autonomy is that the quality of personal decisions may improve as a result of making more of them. Thus, autonomy should be granted, even when it might make things worse in the short term (e.g., letting adolescents making their own decisions), because it will improve people's decision-making ability in the long term.

A third utilitarian advantage is that some people may value autonomy for its own sake, as a fundamental value. What starts out as (or what is most easily justified as) a means value (such as money) can become fundamental.

Note that influence—as opposed to true limitation of choice—affects only the first reason. If you let your teenage daughter buy her own clothes, you can still offer your opinion, and she still gets the learning benefit of making her own choices and listening (or not listening) to others. Such opinions are common enough that it is good to learn to deal with them.

Thus, influence might be harmful if it leads people to make decisions that are different from those they would otherwise make. (And, if it didn't do this, it would be a waste of time for the person trying to do it.) But influence, such as TV programs about small families, is necessarily weak, on the average. Thus, if it switches a decision, the utility loss is necessarily small (unless the influence is accompanied by some implicit threat, such as withdrawal of love or material resources). If people are easily influenced by noncoercive persuasion, then they are unlikely to have had strong preferences from the outset. If there is some counter-vailing benefit to the influence, such as a benefit to the national economy (hence to others), the overall utility may be increased despite the small loss to those who are influenced.

In the case of children, the loss from influence might even be smaller, because the influence may affect people's goals themselves. Thus they somewhat replace themselves with different people, people with slightly different goals—such as wanting two children instead of four.

6.3   Coercion

The situation is different with true coercion. But what is coercion? Faced with a population growth rate that was holding back development, the Chinese government instituted a policy of population control based on material incentives. Families with one child got access to health benefits, schooling, and other social services, which were denied to those with two or more children. Is this coercion?

It may help to look at true coercion, which has also happened in China. Women have been threatened with physical injury in order to force them to have abortions.[1] Where does China's incentive program fit on the scale between soap operas about small families and physical threats?

---

[1]This was not a matter of government policy, except that local officials were rewarded for keeping the birth rate low and often not closely supervised about how they accomplished this.

When we think about incentives, we are subject to framing effects. If we think of the reference point as "full social services," then denial of those services is a harm to large families. If we think of the reference point as "no social services" (as the term "incentive" leads us to do), then we can think of the program as a benefit for small families.

Utility, however, has no natural reference point. Utility theory tells us to think about differences only, and the difference is the same. Moreover, the social services provided are in limited supply. Families cannot be provided more without taking something comparable away from other families. If everyone is to get the same level of health care as those who now qualify for the "incentive," then China will need more doctors and nurses. And the people who become doctors and nurses will have to not do something else, whatever it is, so some production will surely be lost. Or else the level of care will have to decline somewhat for all.

In such situations, there is, of course, an optimum level of inequality, and it might even be zero. The same argument applies to other goods, such as personal income. We use income to encourage people to work; if you don't work then you get paid a lot less. We could create too much inequality or too little. If we do it too much, we will create unnecessary poverty. Too little, and people will work less and be less productive of goods and services that benefit others. Likewise, China's policy may be causing more harm than is warranted by the gains in population control, or it could be about right. (I assume it is not too little, as it has been quite successful in reducing the birth rate.)

But tinkering with the optimum is a choice among options near the "flat maximum" (section 6.2). To a first approximation, giving more money or social services to some and taking the same amount from others is a wash. The utility losses and gains are about equal.

This situation is absent in true coercion. True coercion imposes, or threatens to impose, a "deadweight loss," a loss without anything close to a compensating gain to others. When a woman is beaten for not having an abortion, what she loses cannot be given to anyone else.

Punishment is coercion. The law turns to coercive punishment because it is cheaper to punish people for committing crimes than it is to offer them positive incentives (bribes?) *not* to commit crimes. We can create a large difference in utility for one person—the one who is punished—without much utility loss for anyone else. When used this way, each punishment is a net loss, but the institution of punishment may have overall benefits in the reduction of crime. Thus, coercion can be useful.

Coercion is not useful, however, when people are free to leave the situation in which it is applied, without loss. If we coerce a subject into medical experiments, we can expect people to avoid the situations in which coercion occurs. Thus, it is somewhat self-defeating.

More importantly, though, coercion can cause a large net loss of utility in a way that incentives cannot. If we coerce people into medical experiments (assuming they don't catch on and find a way to avoid us), we could coerce them into experiments whose benefits do not outweigh the costs that result from the coercion. If, on the other hand, we insist that subjects be paid with an incentive, the provision of the incentive itself will cost the researchers about as much as the subjects gain from it. Thus, such incentives will be restricted to cases in which the expected benefit of the research is sufficient so that someone is willing to cover the cost.

Notice, though, that this is almost as far as utilitarianism can go in condemning coercion. But notice also that coercion is already widely employed as a research tool. Some countries have laws about responding to the census. In such cases, coercion—that is, the threat of punishment— is used to enforce participation in data gathering, on the grounds that the social benefits outweigh the resulting costs. Note also that such cases are the result of deliberation by a legislature, not the decision of individual researchers who might be tempted to harm others in order to get their work done more easily.

In sum, coercion does differ from incentives because it involves dead-weight loss. Although coercion sometimes maximizes utility, even for research (the census), the use of coercion involves risks. The requirement that research be "paid for," makes it more likely that the expected benefits of the research outweigh the costs. And by limiting coercive power to government rather than to individuals, we protect people from the self-serving misjudgments of individuals.

There is one more situation in which we may speak of coercion in a sense that can decrease total utility, specifically, when some group uses its influence to change the "reservation payoff" of those who are then coerced (Basu 2002). The reservation payoff is the alternative to entering into an apparently voluntary agreement, such as a subject accepting risk for money. This agreement may be voluntary, given the fact that the subject is very poor and needs the money very badly, for example, for medicine. But suppose the researchers successfully lobby against a program to provide free medical care for the population of interest on the grounds that it would subvert their experiment. In this case, the researchers are using their influence to make the alternative to participation worse than what it would otherwise be. This is actually an example of ordinary coercion as I have defined it, except that the reservation payoff is lowered for an entire group, not just for those who are asked to participate and refuse. Of course, this sort of situation arises elsewhere, for example, when business owners lobby to keep wages and benefits low for the population that provides their workers.

Likewise, when prisoners are promised early release if they participate in research, they are still being coerced by their imprisonment. Again, the relevant definition of coercion is independent of any reference points defined by the status quo or by a default option.

6.4   Research on people who cannot consent

For three years in the mid-1990s, researchers in the United States could not do research on treatments for people coming in to emergency rooms with, for example, strokes, head injuries, or heart attacks. At the time of their admission, such patients were at best semiconscious, and hence incapable of giving informed consent to any experimental treatments (Karlawish, in press). Before this moratorium, emergency research had shown the benefits of "clot busting" drugs for heart attacks, and it had also failed to find benefits of other procedures that were considered promising, such as hypothermia for head injuries. The number of beneficial treatments that was delayed by the moratorium, and the number of patients who died or suffered long-term disability as a result, has apparently not been estimated.[2]

The moratorium was imposed because the legal, or "ethical," basis for the research had become unclear. Researchers had been stretch-

---

[2]Similar problems have occurred in research on children, albeit not so dramatically; see Entorf, Feger, and Kölch (2004).

ing various provisions of the current law that dealt with "deferred consent," waivers for investigational new drugs (which were not always involved), and "minimal risk." The conditions for these provisions were, of course, defined in imprecise language that was supposed to imply sharp cutoffs. The United States regulators decided that the language did not justify what researchers had been doing, which was essentially not obtaining consent when patients were admitted in a state that left them incapable of consenting, for example, unconscious. In October 1996, the United States Department of Health and Human Services issued new regulations that allowed IRBs to approve emergency research (U.S. Department of Health and Human Services 1996). The major criteria are as follows (adapted from Karlawish 2003):

- Necessity requirement: evidence supports the need to do the research, and the subjects are the only population that could reasonably participate in the research.

- Informed consent from the subjects or the subjects' legally authorized representative is not practical.

- Risk-benefit assessment: the research is "potentially beneficial" to the subjects.

- Engagement of the community of potential subjects at the beginning and close of the research: the community of potential subjects has input into the research design and conduct to determine its social worth and learns about the research results.

The researchers still had to try to obtain consent after the fact, and the research was subject to continuing review. The new rules allowed research to go forward, but apparently the additional requirements involved, compared to those in other countries, slowed down research in the United States (Nichol et al. 2003), to the detriment of patients who might benefit from it.

Of course, when criteria are stated in these sorts of legal terms, borderline cases will arise. For example, what does "not practical" mean? or "the community"? or "potentially beneficial"? Often it is not absolutely impossible to obtain consent from family. Rather, such an effort will slow down the administration of the treatment, possibly reducing its beneficial effect. Such a reduction, in turn, could lead researchers to believe that the treatment's benefits were less than they would really be if the treatment were approved for standard use. If it were approved, it could be given immediately. There is a trade-off here between consent and scientific value. In some cases, IRBs have decided that advanced informed consent was possible, because the patient population was already in the hospital (and, e.g., the research concerned methods of emergency resuscitation), but this requirement drastically slowed down the research. Another trade-off is cost. Obtaining consent takes staff time, hence money.

As Karlawish (in press) puts it, "The concept of emergency research is a controversial judgment because it suggests that the interests of subjects —informed consent—can be traded off in the name of efficiency and the interests of society." This was the problem seen by IRBs. The trouble is that informed consent was seen as an absolute, a criterion protected from trade-offs with other criteria. But decision analysis would not look at it this way. It would, instead, ask why informed consent matters, in terms of consequences. It is a means, not an end.

Smithline and Gerstle (1998) asked emergency room patients about whether they approved of a waiver of informed consent. Most of them did, but some did not. About half did not approve if there was a small risk from the treatment under study. The article does not include the wording of the survey used, and, surely, the wording will influence the answers. It isn't even clear whether the question is the correct one to ask. A better question might involve a veil of ignorance (see section 6.5.3): Would you prefer to go to an emergency room that studies new treatments on patients who are unable to consent, or to one that does research only when consent is obtained? Even here, the patients' beliefs about the general benefits of research participation for themselves and others would be relevant. A judgment made on the basis of incorrect beliefs is a good candidate to be overridden by a paternalistic decision (Baron 1996a; see also section 6.7).

The issue of emergency consent raises general questions about why informed consent is needed. I shall return to this issue after a broader discussion.

6.5 Why consent?

The requirement for obtaining consent is often justified in terms of deontological principles such as autonomy and respect for persons. It can also be justified in terms of the economic principle of "Pareto optimality," in combination with the assumption that people are rational in pursuing their interests. A state involving several people is said to be Pareto optimal if nobody can be made better off without making someone else worse off. A transaction leads to a Pareto-optimal state if it makes at least one person better off and nobody worse off. This kind of transaction is a Pareto improvement.

The requirement that a transaction be Pareto optimal is based on consequences, like utilitarianism, but it is more difficult to meet. Any transaction that leads to a Pareto improvement also leads to an increase in total utility, but it is possible to increase total utility by making someone worse off and someone else much better off, and this is not a Pareto improvement. Because Pareto improvements are more conservative, they are often endorsed by those who are reluctant to endorse utilitarianism, with its requirement that the gains for some are comparable to the losses for others. The free market is justified by such an argument, if we assume that people know their own good. Market transactions improve the situation for at least one of those involved, for example, the buyer or seller of a good. And, if both agree and both are rational in pursuing their interests, then we can be sure that nobody is worse off.

Note that "interest" here is *ex ante*, before the outcomes of risks are known. Thus, you may rationally consent to a risky procedure if you think, on balance that the risks are worth taking. You may, in the end, wind up worse off than if you had not agreed to have taken the risk, but your decision may still be rational, and still a Pareto improvement at the time you made it.

Consent is not the only way to insure Pareto improving transactions. Many things we do to people can be assumed not to make them worse off, especially if we assume they are rational. For example, giving rational people a new option without removing any options cannot make them worse off. They don't have to take it. The same rationality assumption is involved here as in the argument for consent—namely, that people make decisions in their own interest. Similarly, we may remove an option but replace it with one that "dominates" the one removed.[3] That is, the new option is better in some ways and worse in no ways. For example, we could reduce the cost of a product but keep everything else the same, or reduce the side effects of a drug, or improve its effectiveness.

The only cases in which we cannot be sure that we are improving matters are those that involve a trade-off, in which at least one dimension is made worse while others are better. We might, for example, increase the price of a drug and improve its effectiveness. Some people might care a lot about the price. They might be stretched to the limit of what they can pay, so they would be harmed by the change, unless the old drug were retained as an option for them. In such cases, consent to switch to the new drug (assuming rationality) insures that the trade-off is indeed beneficial. Research, of course, is often (but not always) in this category. Research has risks that are different in kind from its benefits, so that some people may rationally care more about avoiding the risks than about getting the benefits.

What if some trade-off across dimensions was involved, but we could be sure that all rational people would regard a transaction as not making them worse off. For example, suppose I want to test a drug on you that will increase your life expectancy by five to twenty years (the research question being how many exactly) but will give you a headache for half an hour right after you take it. It is theoretically possible that someone would regard a headache as worse than losing an additional five to twenty years, but it is difficult to imagine. Even someone committed to the Pareto principle might say that consent was unnecessary for this research.

The difficulty increases with the probability that someone would actually be made worse off. As we lower the life expectancy and increase the duration of the headache, we would eventually reach such a point. After reaching this point, a strict Pareto criterion would imply that consent is required from everyone.

---

[3]The idea of dominance is, in essence, Pareto optimality applied to dimensions rather than to people. Both terms may be used for both cases, but I shall stick with the way I've used them here.

6.5.1 A simple decision analysis

A utilitarian criterion, however, would not imply that such consent is required. It would instead compare the expected utility of the available policy options. Here are the main options for a research study:

Enroll All: Enroll everyone in the study.
Consent All: Ask everyone for consent.
Subgroup In: Ask a subgroup for consent, and enroll the rest.
Subgroup Out: Ask a subgroup for consent, and exclude the rest.
Ideal: Ask an all-knowing genie what is best for each person.
Nobody: Exclude everyone.

First let us consider the strategies without the subgroup: Enroll All; Consent All; Ideal; and Nobody. Suppose, for simplicity, that there are two types of people—those who would gain and those who would lose, on the whole, from enrolling. Everyone knows his respective type, so the gainers would consent and the losers would not consent. Let us also assume that Nobody has 0 utility, and the other utilities are relative to this baseline. We need the following quantities:

$$C \quad \text{cost of asking for consent for each person}$$
$$Pg \quad \text{proportion of people who are gainers}$$
$$Ug \quad \text{utility for gainers}$$
$$Ul \quad \text{disutility for losers (a positive number)}$$

Then the utility per person for the other options is as follows:

Enroll All: $(Pg)(Ug) - (1 - Pg)(Ul)$
Consent All: $(Pg)(Ug) - C$
Ideal: $(Pg)(Ug)$

The first two lines imply that the choice of whether to ask anyone for consent or enroll everyone depends on whether $(1 - Pg)(Ul)$ is greater or less than C. Note that $1 - Pg$ is the proportion of losers. Note also that the maximum of Enroll All and Consent All could be less than 0, in which case the study should not be done.

Now suppose that we can select a subgroup of people to ask for consent and either exclude everyone else (Subgroup Out) or include them

(Subgroup In) without asking for consent. To simplify the situation, assume that the selected group and the other group differ only in the probability of being gainers, not in the utility of the gain or loss. Define the following quantities:

Ps proportion of subjects in the subgroup
Pgs proportion of gainers in the subgroup
Pgt proportion of gainers outside of the subgroup

Assume that $Pgs > Pgt$.[4] Then, the expected utility per person for Subgroup In is, $(Ps)(Pgs)(Ug) + (1 - Ps)[(Pgt)(Ug) - (1 - Pgt)(Ul)] - (Ps)(C)$, and for Subgroup Out it is, $(Ps)(Pgs)(Ug) - (Ps)(C)$.

We could imagine other states of affairs. For example, we could suppose that we could perfectly select those who would benefit (but not those who would be harmed) or vice versa. And we could assume that Ug and Ul are different for different subgroups. But the initial point may be clear. There are trade-offs here. In particular, if Consent All and Enroll All were the only two strategies, then the balance between them would depend on whether the cost of obtaining consent is greater than the expected disutility for those mistakenly enrolled if everyone is enrolled. The cost could be quite high if it includes the cost in delay of the research.

The kind of analysis I have just described could be carried out by estimating the relevant quantities, or it could serve as a guide to the way we think less formally about the problem of consent.

This sort of analysis raises two additional major issues. One is the possibility that people are not rational, or not well informed. Then, the models would have to be expanded to include terms for errors made by the subjects themselves (or their surrogates), just in the conditions in which they are asked for consent. These errors would reduce the expected utility of obtaining consent; they would reduce the utility of Consent All relative to all other strategies, and they would reduce the utility of Subgroup In and Subgroup Out relative to Enroll All and Nobody.

The second major issue is the possibility that people will place a value on consent itself. We could incorporate this into the model by assuming different utilities and disutilities for the same outcomes, as a function of

---

[4]For purposes of comparison, note that $Pg = (Ps)(Pgs) + (1 - Ps)(Pgt)$.

whether they came about through getting consent. Or it may be simpler just to include this in the cost term, as a way of reducing the cost (possibly making the cost negative, hence the benefit of asking positive on the whole despite the time and money required). A great deal of psychological literature (e.g., Tyler 1994 and articles cited there) indicates that people are happier with outcomes when they have a voice, even when outcomes are negative.

6.5.2   The utility of consent

But, is this real utility? Should it be counted? There are several different values (and pseudo-values) for informed consent:

- People could have *fundamental values* for being consulted on decisions that affect them (section 3.4). They could value this consultation for its own sake, even if they knew that it would not affect the option chosen, or that it would not improve the expected utility of the option chosen.

- People could have a *means value* (section 3.4). Consent could help to achieve other fundamental values, in particular, the costs and benefits of research in terms of health and money. People may think that the opportunity to give consent insures that these values will be served. They may or may not be correct. At issue here is how good they are as judges of their own good as opposed to how good the researchers are. Surely, the answer depends a lot on who the subjects and researchers are, and the details of the study. Arguably, means values alone are not of concern in a decision analysis. People would want others to attend to their fundamental values whenever they are incorrect about the best decision from that perspective (Baron 1996a). (If they are correct in their means values, there is no distinction in the recommended decision.)

- People have reason to want each other to make good decisions, and one way to promote good decision making is to give people the opportunity to make decisions for themselves, even at the risk of making bad decisions. Thus, informed consent has an *educational value*. This is, in fact, a type of means value.

- People could also have a *moralistic value* (section 3.1.4) for the behavior of asking for consent. They might want researchers to do it, regardless of whether others wanted the same thing, and regardless of whether it had a net benefit when evaluated by nonmoralistic values alone.

- Finally, the preference for giving consent could arise from no value at all but, rather, an *opinion* about what to do. True values for events depend on the events themselves, whether or not they are under any particular person's control. Opinions, however, depend on the existence of a choice that someone must make, such as those who write the laws about informed consent, or researchers. Opinions are typically based on values, but they need not be rationally aligned with all values of the people who have them. Opinions could change through reflection, without any change in fundamental values. In this regard, opinions are like means values.

6.5.3 Measuring the utility of consent

Suppose we wanted to measure the utility of consent, informed by the analysis of the last section. We would carry out some sort of survey of the population of interest. What questions would we ask of our subjects?

We might begin by adopting a "self only" principle advocated in cost-benefit analysis, specifically, that we want to measure each subject's value for herself giving consent, not her altruistic (or moralistic) value for others. In any trade-off between cost and risk, the subject may attempt to guess at the values of others. If subjects guess correctly on the average, then the conclusion of the survey will be the same as if each subject had answered for herself. If, on the other hand, subjects systematically overvalue cost or risk to others, the conclusion may end up being worse for each individual than the result of averaging individual judgments (Jones-Lee 1992). For example, if each subject thinks that everyone else is more concerned about safety than the subject is, measures will be adopted in which people pay more (through taxes, higher cost of drugs, or whatever) for extra safety than it is worth to them.

The self-only principle does not rule out moralistic values (section 3.1.4). Moralistic values are not the same as guesses about what others want, and they may conflict with such guesses. On the other hand, moralistic values concern the behavior of others, not their desires. The only behavior at issue is that of the researchers. Indeed, that is the question at hand. What should the researchers do?

At this point we must distinguish two closely related questions. One is a question about opinion: What should the researchers do? The other is about personal values: What does it mean to you if the researchers do X rather than Y? The second question is the relevant one. The first is not a value but an attempt to second-guess the analysis.

To ask the second question, we could (in principle) say something like: "Suppose that, in one day, you learn that the researchers have decided to do X rather than Y, and you learn that you have just won $1,000 in a lottery. On the whole, would these two events improve your day over what it would have been without either event? Or would they make it worse? Or the same?" We could then vary the amount of money to discover the trade-off between the moralistic value in question and money. Of course, people would have a very hard time answering questions like this, but the point is that, if they understood the question as it is literally intended, measurement is possible. It is a research project in its own right to discover how to help people give honest answers to questions that measure moralistic values.

The means value of consent for achieving health and wealth, is not something we need to ask of our subjects. We do need to know their trade-off between health and wealth. Although the discovery of this trade-off is a difficult problem in practice, it is simpler in principle. Part of the practical difficulty, it should be said, is the fact that money and health have different values to different people. Sometimes those who pay are not the same ones who benefit with better health. In particular, the poor have a higher utility for money than the rich, and also a lower utility for health, given that they are more limited in what they can do with health in a state of poverty.[5]

The means value for education is a different matter. Ideally, we would need to know how beneficial it is for people to live in a society that

---

[5]More generally, we can think of the money-health trade-off as involving length of life, which is affected mainly by health, various dimensions of quality of life, which differ in the extent to which they are sensitive to money or health, and, in addition, value for posterity, which is affected mainly by money.

is a little more encouraging of individual decision making. There is a continuum here. Even communist governments allowed autonomy in some areas of life (marriage, for example), while the most laissez-faire governments—which tend to be the weakest governments rather than those that support market economies (which require restrictions concerning property rights, contracts, and so forth)—manage to impose some constraints, if only through vigilante justice. So when we examine whether some particular area of life should have more or less individual control, we must view this on the background of what is already present in a given society. It is extremely difficult to examine this issue empirically. I know of few studies that have even attempted it. (Cross-national studies usually have many other confounded variables.)

In such a situation, we must rely on what Keeney (1992) calls a proxy value, a type of means value. We cannot estimate the true effect of interest, so we rely on some other measure that is related to it. For example, if we are interested in the value of reducing air pollution, we really want to know its effects on health and the natural environment, but these effects are so complex that we might resort to asking experts how much they value reducing pollution by X particles per cubic meter. Similarly, in the case of autonomy, we might simply ask people how much good they think it does (compared to some suitable alternative dimension).

Some people might be tempted to answer in terms of the precedent value of a particular decision. "Once we take away personal choice in this area," they may think, "we will go down a slippery slope, and soon we will have a paternalistic dictatorship." The trouble with slippery slopes is that they could go either way. We could go down a slope toward anarchy as well. And the political process often works to correct excesses in either direction, making the slopes less slippery. When there is a happy medium, one way to reach it is to make case by case decisions about what is better for the case at hand—more autonomy or less. Such a practice also sets a precedent for always making the best decision, which is not a bad precedent to set. Thus, I would argue that we should exclude slippery-slope beliefs from elicitation of values and ask people to focus on the case at hand as if it would affect no other future decisions of the same type. Again, subjects will have difficulty following this instruction, but at least it is meaningful.

What I have argued here is that it is possible in principle to do a decision analysis of informed consent in emergency research. I'm not sure such an analysis is worth doing numerically. The elements of error in the analysis are so great that it would surely lead to erroneous decisions. But the decision analysis, if it could be done, is the right way to make the decision, in terms of insuring the best outcomes. Any other method, such as the traditional bioethical method of intuitively balancing principles and devising a flowchart, is surely just as error prone—or more—by the same criterion. If we attempt to keep in mind this kind of analysis when crafting rules for research, it calls our attention to relevant issues.

For me, in the case of emergency research, I would try to avoid anything that would impair the research itself. I would not want to die, or suffer permanent disability, because some research did not get done that could have saved me, because the consent procedures were slowing down the research. In return for this, I would happily forgo the option to consent to emergency research that was thought to be reasonable by others, even if some of the research had a negative expected utility. I would hope that those who do, and approve, such research would make sure that, on balance, the total set of research studies done had a positive expected utility for the subjects. Although politically I tend toward the libertarian view that autonomy should be increased, I do not see emergency research as a good candidate for such a change.[6] I believe my preference here (and that is all it is) is typical of people in most of the developed world.

My little personal exercise here suggests how researchers or their overseers might decide what kind of consent should be used. It is a form of the "veil of ignorance" (Rawls's 1971 [section 24] term), but used, as Harsanyi (1953) did, as part of a utilitarian approach. The idea is to ask what decision you would make without knowing who you are, assuming that you have an equal chance to become each person affected. This is not so difficult to imagine in cases like the ones at issue here, since practically everyone might become an emergency patient.

---

[6]Better candidates might be: the freedom to contractually forgo the right to sue the sellers of goods or services, including health care, in return for lower prices; and the freedom to take recreational drugs, with adequate information about their risks.

6.6   Altruism, hope, and consent

In some ways, the main contribution of modern bioethics is its emphasis on informed consent (Wikler 1994). A second principle is that it is wrong to harm some in order to help others.

These two principles play out together strangely when it comes to research on human subjects. Most IRBs do not allow researchers to tell subjects much, if anything, about the potential benefits of a study for future patients. One idea, apparently, is that researchers would exude optimism and falsely entice altruistic subjects into participation. This position is difficult to maintain, since researchers have the same temptation to minimize the risks of the study when recruiting subjects, yet they are allowed to try to present the risks accurately. Another possible justification of this exclusion is that IRBs believe that altruism should not be a motive for participation. For many studies, however, exclusion of altruism would leave no rational motive at all: subjects are unlikely to benefit from experiments that do not involve therapeutic agents, for example.

Thus, in the typical consent form given to subjects, they are told of the risks but not the benefits. They must consent, and they must be scrupulously informed. Yet one piece of information is typically withheld, namely, the potential benefit of the research for others. Subjects in drug trials, for example, are rarely told whether the drug being tested is promising. They are not told what kind of evidence about related drugs or animal studies led to the current research. It is as if the withholding of this information removes the possibility that the researcher will put some at risk for the benefit of others.

The same information is usually relevant to the subjects' hope for benefit for themselves. If a new drug is promising although risky, it is more rational to take the risk than if the drug is a long shot. Yet, researchers are usually prevented from telling potential subjects about promise, lest the researchers exaggerate and induce the subjects to take more risk than they would rationally take. This is a crude solution at best.

One problem is that this procedure ignores the subjects' altruism. They may be willing to put themselves at risk. But if they are at all conflicted about this—and reasonable people cannot have unlimited altruism—they should know how much good is expected in return for how much risk. Technically, this is part of what I called U in the last section, the utility of participation in a research study for those correctly included. But it might be worth separate consideration.

Perhaps another justification for prohibiting the mention of benefits to others is that some subjects would see it as a kind of pressure. If these benefits were mentioned, potential subjects might feel that they were being asked to be altruistic. It is possible that appeals to altruism that also involve risk could lead people into commitments that they come to regret. Perhaps the resulting disutility would outweigh the increased utility from having more subjects, especially when we consider the effect of such regret, when it becomes known to other potential subjects, on future recruitment. This is an empirical question.

On the other hand, the role of altruism could be an example of the flat maximum (section 6.2). Subjects may be nearly indifferent if their altruism is just enough to induce them to participate. An appeal to their altruism could lead them to violate, in some sense, their true values. But the violation would be small because they were close to indifference at the outset. Hence, little harm would be done, in terms of loss of expected utility to them, in return for great possible gain for others.

But, in fact, the withholding of information about altruism or hope for personal benefit probably does not work. Surely potential subjects insert their own hunches. They suspect that researchers cannot tell the truth about the potential benefit to self and others, so the subjects make it up. The result is that subjects make decisions on the basis of random beliefs that have little relation to the best information they could get. Surely, they make avoidable errors: they volunteer for risky studies that are known to have little expected benefit, believing that the researchers are forced not to mention the benefits, when, in fact, the researchers are, for a change, omitting nothing relevant. We have a complex game going on among IRBs, researchers, and subjects, with each trying to second-guess the others. The solution is to legalize honesty.

If subjects were honestly informed, they would be able to evaluate the trade-off between risk and inconvenience to themselves, on the one hand, and benefits to themselves and others, on the other hand. People have limited altruism. They thus consider benefit to others but not without limit. It is difficult to imagine that anyone is a perfect moral utilitarian, weighing himself exactly as much as anyone else and no more.

6.7 Competence to consent

Consent is involved in many decisions—research participation, medical procedures, living wills, release of records, assisted suicide, and so on. Many people are impaired in the cognitive capacities needed to give consent. What should be done about this? A standard practice is to appoint some sort of surrogate for the person concerned. But how do we know when the surrogate is needed, or that the surrogate knows better? And what if the patient disagrees with the surrogate? It is usually not sufficient to make such decisions based on a person's diagnosis, given that most conditions that impair function are matters of degree. There is no sharp cutoff for mental retardation, senile dementia, schizophrenia, psychotic depression, or youth.

The same issues arise for children and adolescents as for adults with diminished capacity, but most legal systems give health professionals much less choice in dealing with young people. Still, it is interesting to ask what the law should be. Thus, I will discuss the issues in the abstract, without considering any particular groups. I think that the major questions apply to all groups.

One common method for assessing competence uses a structured interview that tests the subject's understanding and appreciation of the information presented in the consent form (Appelbaum et al. 1999; Etchells et al. 1999; Fazel, Hope, and Jacoby 1999; Karlawish, Casarett, and James 2002; Kim et al. 2001; see Kim, Karlawish, and Caine 2002, for a review). The answers are scored by raters according to a list of criteria. For example, Appelbaum et al. (1999) used a version of the MacArthur Competence Assessment Tool:

> Questions for assessing understanding focused on 13 pieces of critical information concerning the psychotherapy study's purpose, procedure, benefits, risks, and alternatives (e.g., "What is the purpose of the research project I described to you?"). The three appreciation questions focused on subjects' beliefs about whether what they had been told actually applied to themselves, specifically, 1) "Do you believe that you have been asked to be in this study primarily for your benefit?"; 2) "Do you believe, as part of this study, that you will

see your therapist as often as he/she thinks is best for your care?"; and 3) "What do you believe would happen if you were to decide not to be in this study any longer?" Reasoning questions centered on subjects' abilities to compare research participation with other treatment options and to describe the everyday consequences of participation and nonparticipation (e.g., "What is it that makes [the subject's preferred option] seem better than [the nonchosen options]?").

Typical findings are that these measures do distinguish people who are cognitively impaired (e.g., with Alzheimer's disease or schizophrenia) from those who are not impaired (e.g., the caregivers of the Alzheimer's patients), but the groups overlap. If we score the interview by some sort of point system and apply a cutoff, any cutoff that is low enough so that all of the control group passes will also pass a substantial portion of the impaired group, including many who fail answer some of the basic questions.

6.7.1 Testing good judgment

The tests in question seem to be assessing requirements for decision making rather than good judgment. It might be instructive, though, to ask whether we could construct a test of good judgment. A problem is that it is difficult to find questions about decision making that have correct answers independent of the subject's utilities (values). If we knew, or could assume, a person's utilities, we could construct items that measure whether a person's judgments about what to do are in line with his own values.

For example, we could use the "conjoint analysis" method that is often used in marketing research, in which objects are presented one by one, and the subject makes a judgment of each object on (for example) a scale of desirability from 1 to 7 (see section 3.3). The objects might be research studies, and the dimensions might be rate of pay, chance of side effects, probability of benefit, commuting time, and so on. We could ask whether variation in each dimension affects the judgment appropriately. We could also ask about the subject's consistency or predictability: how much would his judgments vary if the same item were presented at different points in a sequence of many judgments.[7]

We could get around the problem of not knowing the subject's values in several ways. One is to tell the subject what his values are and ask him to make judgments as if he had those values. This tests his ability to translate values into judgments, but the test is also affected by his ability to understand and use what is communicated to him—perhaps even the difficulty of putting aside his own values. One way to communicate values to the subject is to ask him to predict how someone else would respond. The subject would see how the other person responds, then get feedback about his answers.

Another way to test the subject is to ask him to predict the average person's responses. The domain could be selected so that people do not differ much. Thus, the subject's ability to make reasonable, typical decisions could be assessed.

How could we score a test like this so that the score would be useful? The most direct way, I think, is to estimate the total utility if all the subject's judgments were turned into decisions, and then compare that to the maximum total utility possible if the subject made perfect judgments in line with the given values. For example, if the judgments were on a 7-point scale, we could look at all the possible pairs of judgments that the subject made and assume that, when the ratings differed, he would choose the option with the higher rating. (And, for ties, we could assume that each option would be chosen equally often.) Since we know the utilities, we could calculate the utility of each choice, compared to the best choice.

We would then get a utility-loss score for each subject. How could we decide how much loss is enough to take away the person's decision making power? (Let us put aside the educational benefits of allowing people to make their own decisions. This matters most in the case of children, but they are the ones most limited by law.)

We need to compare the loss in utility to that arising from the alternatives. One alternative is to appoint a surrogate who knows the decision maker. Even such a surrogate may fail to make choices in line with the

---

[7]We could also infer this variability by fitting a model to the subject's judgments and looking at the error in the model's predictions.

actual subject's values. Another alternative is to use some sort of default choice determined by a panel of judges.

These alternatives have two sources of error of their own. One is that they may rely on values different from those of the subject in question. For the default choice, such errors will result from individual differences in values. The greater the individual differences, the greater the utility loss from failing to take them into account. The surrogate ought to do somewhat better in this regard, but a single surrogate is likely to be more error prone for the same reason that anyone is error prone: it is just difficult to make consistent judgments (Dawes, Faust, and Meehl 1989).

Studies of the effectiveness of surrogates (e.g., Coppolino and Ackerson 2001) usually look at the number of cases of disagreement in which the surrogate is asked to predict the decision maker's actual decision, especially false positives in which the surrogate says yes but the decision maker says no. False positives occur. What we do not know is how serious they are. If, of course, we take a kind of absolutist, legalistic view that any false positive is terrible, seriousness does not matter. But it does for utility. We need to look at the utility loss that results from errors, not just their presence. And there will be false positive (and false negative) errors both ways: those resulting from appointing a surrogate, and those resulting from failing to appoint one. Thus, we cannot avoid errors. To compare one method of making decisions to another, we need to ask about the cost of errors, not just their presence.

In sum, from a utilitarian point of view, the real issue is the potential loss of utility resulting from bad decisions. It seems not all that difficult to measure this loss, at least approximately. There are clear trade-offs, between tailoring decisions to the individual and error in judgment itself.

6.7.2   What matters?

Instead of presenting a subject with all the details, we could lead her through a decision analysis of whether to participate in the research (or have the surgery, or whatever). Although such a process sounds more complicated, it might actually be simpler. Most of what is presented in the usual consent procedure is irrelevant to most people. It might not be so bad at all if the subject were unable to recall the various elements included in current tests of competence.

For what it is worth, if I were asked to read (or listen to) a consent form without knowing that I would be tested on it, I would surely fail any assessment based on the MacArthur Competence Assessment Tool. I would simply not pay attention to facts that did not concern me. For example, if I suspect (as I do) that researchers do not mean it when they say that there is no benefit, I would both expect and ignore that part, and I would not remember it. If I had had blood drawn before, I would neither listen to nor recall the particular list of risks of a blood draw that the researchers included in this particular consent form. Conversely, if I understood that some risks that were especially serious for me, or (more likely) that the research was time consuming and the pay insufficient, I would not pay attention to anything else. Although the official idea of a consent procedure is that the subject should attend to everything, understand it, and remember it, such thoroughness is rarely needed in the real world. Subjects should not be declared incompetent because they can distinguish what is relevant from what is not, or because they trust researchers.

Instead, it would make sense to do research to find out how individuals actually differ, and use this information to decide what to ask patients (as suggested by Nease and Owens 1994, in the context of decision analysis recommendations rather than consent). If individuals do not differ much, then it may not serve any purpose to ask consent at all, aside from the psychological benefits for the subject or patient. In other cases, researchers can find out where the real differences are, and find where each patient or subject stands on the continua that actually matter. For example, decisions about fetal testing for Down syndrome seem to hinge largely on the value for avoiding Down versus that for avoiding a miscarriage or abortion (Kupperman et al. 1999, 2000). Or utility of angina symptoms may vary considerably and largely determine whether bypass surgery is warranted (Nease et al. 1995).

Consent could be much easier if the consent procedure focused on what really mattered. By putting aside what was irrelevant or assumed, patients or subjects might find it easier to focus on the relevant dimensions. They would not need to recall details that did not matter to them in order to be assumed competent. Even in this case, however, we can ask whether impaired groups make sufficient errors in expressing their judgments so that surrogates would do a better job, even though surrogates would probably not represent patients values as well as the patients themselves. These are all empirical questions. But in the absence of research that attempts to answer them, at least the questions focus us on what is relevant in making decisions about who should be asked.

6.7.3   Can poor decisions indicate incompetence?

I have often heard people say that some patient decisions are so irrational that they indicate incompetence by their nature and should thus be overridden. A patient who refuses treatment because he hears voices telling him that his doctors are trying to poison him is clearly showing psychotic symptoms. The refusal was just the occasion to manifest them. The same might be true if the voices tell him that God will punish him for taking the medicine. But what if God told him that God will cure the disease only if he refuses treatment? Or what if his personal religion holds that life is in God's hands? Or what if it is an organized religion such as Christian Science, which prohibits many medical interventions? The problem is that the line between unusual beliefs and psychotic delusions is not sharp. Moreover, the beliefs that are unusual at one time may predominate at another time. Even some conspiracy theories are true.

One might think that the opportunity for going against the patient's true values is greater when her competence is judged from her decision in the case at hand rather than when it is judged from some sort of test. But the opposite could be true. The generality of mental tests is often poor. A person can be generally insane yet able to make some decisions quite rationally, and a generally sane person could have a particular domain of extreme irrationality. Moreover, judgments of rationality are never free from bias if the person making the judgment has an interest in saying that the subject is irrational. If we are worried about such bias, we can try to have some disinterested party make the judgment. Or a less expensive alternative is for those involved to make the judgment on the basis of documented evidence that could be examined by others in case of a challenge, such as a tape-recorded interview.

6.8   Responsibility and the law

Bad things occasionally happen to research subjects and patients. Doctors and researchers make mistakes. Sometimes a side effect appears that was not anticipated. Sometimes things happen right after an experiment that seem to be related to the experiment but are not. When such things happen, the law often enters the picture. The relevant law is usually not the criminal law but the law of torts.

Tort law itself may be understood in utilitarian terms (e.g., Kaplow and Shavell 2002; Shavell 1987). Consider a case in which a research subject is injured in an experiment. Who is responsible? For a start, consider the case in which the harm is monetary. Thus, we can ask whether the experimenter or the subject should pay for the loss.

The law-and-economics tradition looks at the consequences of this decision. The main consequences are the incentive provided for others in the same situation. The case is an example of a class of similar cases treated the same way. If the experimenter pays, then other experimenters, knowing that they would have to pay too, have an incentive to take care. In fact, the incentive they have is enough so that the extra (marginal) cost of additional care is just greater than the expected cost of additional harm (taking into account the probability). For example, if the probability of losing $100,000 is one in ten thousand, and the expected cost of preventing this loss is $11, the expenditure is not worth it. Better to take the risk of loss and pay those subjects who suffer loss. This way, total cost is minimized. If the experimenter took more care than this, her costs would be more than the benefits in terms of the harm prevented. (Remember, the harm is monetary.)[8]

On the other hand, if the law says that the experimenter is not responsible, then the subject must pay. The incentive effect of such a requirement is that other subjects will take additional care. They will read the consent form more carefully, and perhaps stay away from some experiments.

What should the rule be? Who should pay? The issue, according to this analysis, hinges on the question of who can reduce the risk most

---

[8]This analysis ignores the possibility that the utility of money is greater for the subject than for the experimenter. This neglect is a simplification.

efficiently, what Calabresi (1970) called the "least cost avoider." If the law makes experimenters pay to reduce the risk, and if subjects could reduce the risk more cheaply, then the payment is inefficient. Of course, the question of who is the least-cost avoider depends on what the next step is to avoid harm, what additional precaution could be taken by each party. In this case, the cost must be the total cost, including the cost of lost scientific information if the research is not done and the cost in difficulty of recruiting other subjects if a subject is harmed and not compensated.

Tort law has a second function, compensation of those who are injured, the victims. Compensation and incentive are different functions. The utilitarian theory of monetary compensation is that compensation is justified by the fact that injury increases the utility of money. If you lose money, then money has more utility to you than it did before.

In the case of nonmonetary injuries, monetary compensation provides resources to those who can put them to good use—for example, the cost of a medical treatment to fully cure some condition caused by an experiment. When the injurer compensates the victim, as when a child is induced to give back something he has taken or when a victim sues an injurer in court, punishment and compensation are linked, but they need not be linked. Criminals are punished (made to pay) even when they do not compensate their victims, and people are compensated for injuries by insurance.

The justification for compensation is, in fact, the same as that for insurance. Indeed, a scheme of insurance could, in principle, replace the compensation function of tort law. New Zealand has a system something like this, in which tort penalties are paid to the state, not the victim, and compensation for the victim comes from a social insurance plan paid for by the government (using money from penalties as well as taxes). One advantage of this system is that it can provide compensation even when nobody is legally at fault. It also prevents overcompensation, when the victim gets more than needed (in terms of utility maximization) just because deterrence requires a large penalty against the injurer.

The utilitarian theory of monetary compensation is that money becomes more valuable after a loss so that total utility is increased by giving money to those who lose. If you get a bacterial infection, you have a way of spending money to increase your utility that you did not have before the infection. You gain more utility from spending money on antibiotics than you could have gained from any way of spending money beforehand. This is a nonintuitive conclusion, because it implies that utility is not increased by compensation when the utility of money is not increased by the injury, for example, when a child is killed.

The utilitarian analysis of torts sometimes conflicts with our intuitive judgments. When many people think about tort law, they tend to treat all cases as if they were a single standard type in which punishment and compensation are linked and in which the beneficial consequences of punishment are irrelevant. Baron and Ritov (1993) found, for example, that subjects assessed higher tort penalties against an injurer when the injurer paid the victim directly, compared to a situation like that in New Zealand, where the injurer paid the government and the government paid the victim. We found this result even when the penalty had no beneficial deterrent effect (because, for example, the company would stop making a drug rather than take greater care in making it).

Tort penalties have caused highly beneficial products—such as vaccines and birth control products—to be withdrawn and have led to a reduction in research and development expenditures for similar products. For example, production of pertussis vaccine (which, as noted earlier, prevents whooping cough but also causes rare but serious side effects) declined drastically in the United States as a result of lawsuits, and the price increased, until 1986, when Congress passed a law to provide some protection against lawsuits.

These effects may happen because of the intuitions of those involved in the system—judges, lawyers, plaintiffs, defendants, and juries—about what penalties ought to be assessed and what compensation ought to be paid. In particular, two basic intuitive principles may be involved: the desire for retribution against an injurer, whatever the consequences of the retribution; and the feeling that harms caused by people are more deserving of compensation than those caused by nature. These intuitions are not based on expected consequences, so it is not surprising that they sometimes lead to consequences that we find objectionable. (See Baron 1998 for further discussion.)

Because the tort system sometimes "punishes the innocent"—or at least punishes those who are not the least-cost avoiders—fear of lawsuits can lead researchers and health professionals to take excessive care. Consent forms become longer, and consent procedures take more time, so that those involved have a legal defense. The law cannot be trusted either to assign responsibility correctly or to balance the costs and benefits of additional consent procedures themselves. From a utilitarian perspective, this is just an unhappy fact of life. The law itself will hold back the improvement of consent procedures.

6.9   Conclusion

I have argued that consent procedures should be analyzed in terms of their costs and benefits, in utility terms. The usual analysis of consent in terms of principles such as autonomy and competence is often consistent with such utility maximization. In general, autonomy maximizes utility. But rigid application of principles, or the attempt to balance them intuitively, may reduce utility. For example, autonomy may have little value for flat-maximum decisions. Likewise, the attempt to influence a decision may do little harm, and it may have some benefit. Influence is not the same as coercion, even when a decision is completely predictable. The harm from violation of autonomy is largely in the loss of utility that comes from forcing options on people that are much worse than they would choose for themselves. Such harm is unlikely to result from, for example, a researcher telling a potential subject (truthfully) that a study is likely to yield beneficial knowledge.

Likewise, information is valuable because it helps people make better decisions. Too much information can hurt. Even the attempt to get consent itself may be harmful, when the need to obtain consent slows down the research and when consent would be given anyway in good time. Possibly, the testing of gene therapy for ornithine transcarbamylase deficiency (the condition that Jesse Gelsinger had) in infants is an example.

Yet, sometimes "ethics" seems to require researchers to withhold information that is highly relevant, in particular, information relevant to altruistic desires. Altruism is, happily, part of people's good. Why pretend it isn't?

People may differ in their competence to make decisions that maximize their utilities. Incompetence is a problem to the extent that it leads people to choose worse options, and the harm of incompetence is the difference between what is chosen and what is best. Although we may have trouble applying this principle directly, it may at least clarify what we are aiming at in testing or defining competence.

One factor I have not mentioned so far, which will come up in the next chapter, is the interest of researchers and health professionals in their reputations. When these professionals harm their subjects or patients, they reduce their ability to attract new subjects and patients. Some of this reputation effect is individual. An individual doctor can get a bad reputation.

But some of it is more general: researchers in a certain field, or researchers in general, can get a bad reputation and find it difficult to attract subjects. Or, to take another example, if researchers in a certain field get a reputation for deceiving their subjects, the subjects will not believe what researchers tell them. (In my own research, I practice no *active* deception. I do sometimes refrain from telling the subjects about my hypothesis. But subjects sometimes still ask me, "OK, what was that study *really* about?")

Because researchers can often benefit at the expense of their fellow researchers, they have a conflict of interest. That is the topic of the next chapter.

Chapter 7

Conflict of Interest

Conflict of interest arises when agents (which is what I shall call them) hold jobs or positions designed for some purpose, yet they can use their positions to help themselves in ways not intended by the design. Agents often give in to this temptation, without knowing that they are doing so (Bazerman, Morgan, and Loewenstein 1997).

The problem is ubiquitous and serious. One aspect of it is government corruption, which is a major problem that holds back the economic development of many of the world's poorest countries, although corruption is not unknown in the richer countries. Closer to the present topic, physicians have conflicts when they can make money from services they advise their patients to get, or, on the other side, when they are rewarded by insurers for saving money on other services. And researchers have conflicts when they can do their research more easily by neglecting risks to their subjects, or by not disclosing them.

We have several ways of reducing these conflicts or their effects. One is to design institutions that insulate agents from potential conflict. The use of lifetime tenure for teachers, professors, and judges is justified in part by the fact that these agents must make decisions about others (grades, sentences) and should therefore not be subject to threats involving loss of their jobs. Sometimes decisions are subject to review, approval, or appeal, or they must be made public. Or potential influences must be made public. Or they must be secret (such as the decisions of voters) so that reward and punishment cannot be applied by outsiders.

A second method for reducing the effect of conflict is the law. Most serious violations are, in fact, illegal. The problem is that enforcement of the law requires the cooperation of those involved, including the agents themselves. Most corruption is illegal, but law enforcers are themselves part of the corruption, and, besides, violators are usually not reported because the ones who might report them are also violating the law. To some extent, corruption exists because it is expected. It is like an unwritten law that everyone follows because they assume (perhaps correctly) that everyone else follows it and nothing else is expected of them.

Here is where the third method comes in, which is codes of ethics. A good code will attempt to state agents' common practices in a way that is both believable to agents and acceptable to clients—that is, those who are affected by the judgments that agents are supposed to make. It may thus push agents toward greater resistance to temptation, but not so much as to be impossible to follow. It is effective, in part, because it undercuts the justification that weak-willed agents often provide: "Everyone else does this, so why shouldn't I?"

The final method of interest is regulation, which delegates powers to regulatory agencies, such as Institutional Review Boards (IRBs). Such agencies have the power of the law, but they are able to tailor the law to local conditions, insofar as such tailoring is needed.

7.1   Ethics

It is often said that utilitarianism leaves no place for "ethics," except insofar as the word means "morality." I shall argue that codes of ethics have a role that can be justified in utilitarian terms. Namely, they provide a reference point for resolving difficult conflicts between self-interest and the good of others. They make such conflicts easier to resolve.

7.1.1   Why might codes of ethics work

From a utilitarian perspective, agents have some reason to follow a code of ethics, but not much. The general problem is related to the idea of weighted utilitarianism (Baron 1993a, 1997a). The idea of weighted utilitarianism is that perfect utilitarianism is impossibly demanding as a philosophy of personal behavior, because it requires that we weigh our own interests no more than those of anyone else, so we always sacrifice our self-interest whenever we can provide someone else with a greater utility gain than our loss from doing so. As Singer (1993) has argued, this could reduce most of us to poverty. Thus, we adopt a more realistic standard, which is to weigh ourselves more than others but also try to do this consistently, so as to get the largest benefit to others for any given amount of self-sacrifice we are willing to make.

This theory of weighted utilitarianism says less than it may appear to say. (See Baron 2000 for criticisms.) In particular, it is not the answer to the moral question, "What should I do?" It would be better, morally, to make a greater self-sacrifice for others than this theory would ask, for any given personal weight. Nor is it the answer to the question of what is rational for you to do in the pursuit of your own goals. The answer to that depends on the extent to which you are altruistic—that is, the extent to which you have goals for the achievement of others' goals. If you have no altruism, then you achieve your goals best by completely ignoring the goals of others. But the theory still might provide a rough approximation to what codes of ethics are trying to do.

In particular, imagine a graph, such as figure 7.1, in which the horizontal axis is how far you go in denying your self-interest for the benefit of others. Points on this axis are choices, ordered in terms of the ratio of your loss to others' benefit, with the lowest ratio (most benefit to others for a given loss) on the left. Each unit on this axis is a given amount of loss to yourself. (This is artificial. It assumes that each act has the same loss.) Each agent sets a cutoff on this line, performing all actions to the left of the cutoff. The higher the cutoff, the more scrupulous the agent. The vertical axis shows the cumulative benefit to others of performing all the acts up to each cutoff. Up to the cutoff of 30, the benefits to others are ten times the loss to you, so it is worthwhile to go this far, so long as you weigh yourself less than ten times what you weigh others. Beyond 30, the benefits to others are 1.5 times the cost to you. If you go beyond this point, you are weighing others almost as much as yourself.

If such a point existed, at which the benefit/cost ratio declines sharply, it would be reasonable to try to advise everyone to adopt at least this level of stringency. More than this would produce less benefit for a given amount of self-sacrifice. Codes of ethics would lead to a kind of lim-

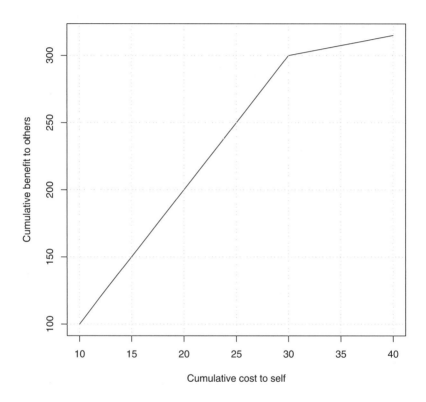

Figure 7.1: Hypothetical benefit/cost function for self-sacrifice

ited utility maximization if they picked this point as the one in the code. Less stringency would mean that more benefits could be achieved for an amount of sacrifice that agents were willing to make. More stringency would entail some loss in efficiency.

It is very doubtful that codes of ethics work this way. More likely, the curve has no sharp corner. The ideal code of ethics would make the best compromise between putting the cutoff too low, so that people who would be willing to be more stringent are encouraged to be more selfish, and putting it too high, so that those who are less stringent do not follow the code. In principle, these losses could both be quantified, so that the ideal point could be determined. The greatest difficulty in practice, I suspect, is in determining the effect of codes on actual behavior.

Psychologically, codes of ethics may work because people are motivated to conform, and the code may convince agents that conformity means following the code. The most relevant evidence comes from the study of social dilemmas. In the most typical form of social dilemma studied in the laboratory, each of several people (typically about 6) has two choices, C (cooperate) and D (defect). All choices are made without knowing what others have chosen. Choice C is worse for the chooser but better for everyone else, compared to D. For example, if you choose C, each of the others will get $1 more than they would each get otherwise, and you will get nothing more; if you choose D, then you will get $1 more and the others will get nothing more. If each dollar has one unit of utility (one utile), then C is best for the group (with 5 extra utiles if there are 6 people), and D is best for you.

In this simple situation, a utilitarian analysis indicates that the benefit of cooperation (C) does not depend on the number of others who also choose C. Each C response does a fixed amount of good for others, with the loss of a fixed amount for you, regardless of what others are doing. Psychologically, though, people seem to think of these situations as if benefits were available only if a sufficient number chose C. Thus, the choice of C is highly correlated with beliefs about whether others will choose C. And, manipulation of this belief by experience has a strong effect on choices (Dawes et al. 1986; Fehr and Gächter 2000; Tyran 2002). People want to do their part if others do their part. It is interesting that this result has little to do with whether the benefit of one's own cooperation depends on the cooperation of others.

This sort of "reciprocity" or "contingent cooperation" may help codes of ethics to work. If people think that others follow the code, they will be motivated to do the same, regardless of the utilitarian costs and benefits.

7.1.2   Intrinsic motivation

Implicit in the last subsection was the assumption that codes of ethics can work, even if they are advisory, because people are motivated to conform to them. There is, in fact, considerable evidence for such intrinsic motivation to "do the right thing." More importantl, such motivation is sometimes undermined by the attempt to impose rules and sanctions (such as those imposed by review boards). The undermining effect is sometimes so large that the attempt to control behavior backfires, so that violations are more likely to occur when they are rigidly controlled than when people are trusted. Putting this another way, trust inspires trustworthiness, and mistrust leads people to live down to expectations.

Intrinsic motivation has been understood for some time (e.g., Lepper and Greene 1978). A couple of recent findings are particularly relevant to conflict-of-interest regulation, the topic of this chapter. Schweitzer and Ho (2004) studied behavior in a repeated trust game. In each play, player A can give player B some money, which doubles in value, and then B can return some of the money to A (possibly just A's contribution, but also possibly a share of the "profit"). The B player was more trustworthy (returned more money) when he knew that the A was monitoring him than when the returns were anonymous. But the monitoring actually led to reduced trustworthiness when B knew that he was not being monitored. On the whole, because there were enough nonmonitoring trials, the monitoring led to reduced trustworthiness overall.

In another study, Cain, Loewenstein, and Moore (2005) argue that rules requiring disclosure of conflict of interest can have a perverse effect on honesty. They asked one subject, an "estimator," to estimate some quantity (the value of a jar of coins) with the advice of second subject, an "adviser," who had more information about the quantity in question. In one condition, the adviser and the estimator were both paid according to the estimator's accuracy. In other conditions, the adviser was paid more when the estimator was too high, thus creating a conflict of interest between the two subjects. In one of these conflict conditions, the adviser disclosed the conflict to the estimator, and, in another, she did not. The adviser actually provided higher estimates in the disclosure condition, and, as a result, the estimator performed worse. The rule requiring disclosure "licensed" the adviser to stretch the truth even more. Again, mistrust undermined trustworthiness.[1]

7.1.3   An example: Deception

Academic disciplines differ in their attitudes toward deception of research subjects. (IRBs, in my experience, typically do not take strong positions on this issue.) Psychology, especially social psychology, has a long history of using deception, for example, using stooges to pose as confederate subjects. Indeed, deception is by some accounts central to social psychology: in order to test the central assumption that people respond to their perception of the social situation rather than to the situation itself, researchers must manipulate that perception, often to the extent of becoming theatrical directors.

On the other side, experimental economics use real, monetary rewards, and they want their subjects to believe that these rewards are truly available. Experimental economists thus regard social psychologists as poisoners of their subject pools who lead potential subjects to believe that experiments often involve deception (Hertwig and Ortman 2001). If anything, social psychologists' efforts to "debrief" their subjects, that is, to explain the deception at the experiment, make things worse by making the expectation of deception even more widespread, although sometimes the debriefing is necessary as an attempt to prevent subjects from having generally false beliefs (especially about themselves). From the economists' perspective, deception is an uncooperative act: It helps the individual researcher who does it, at the expense of other researchers.

As a result of this attitude, experimental economists have created informal codes of research ethics, which they enforce partly by social pressure but also through the process of reviewing grant proposals and journal articles. Some journals will not publish research involving deception.

---

[1]For other studies reinforcing this general conclusion, see: Falk (2004), Fehr and Rockenbach (2003), Frey and Jegen (2001), and Frey Oberholzer-Gee (1997).

A decision analysis of this problem would try to assess the costs and benefits of deception. It would be nice to have data on the effect of researchers' practices on their reputations for telling the truth before experiments. Another issue is the effect of trust on the validity of the conclusions from the research. Finally, it would be nice to know the cost and effectiveness of alternative approaches, such as asking subjects after an experiment whether they believed what they were told, or trying to create local reputations for honesty. ("This is the economics department. We don't deceive people here.") If it turned out that, in a given setting, the presence of psychologists made subjects less trusting of economists, but that the economists could compensate for this by testing more subjects and then excluding the ones who suspect what they were told—but not by developing a local reputation—the economists might reasonably ask the psychologists to compensate them for the extra costs.

Of course, it is difficult to get the relevant data to do this sort of analysis. In the absence of data, any person or group in a situation of authority would have to make judgments about the relevant probabilities and costs. At least, the attempt to make these judgments could reduce the sort of posturing over absolute principles that sometimes occurs in discussions of issues like these.

7.2   Reforming the IRB

IRBs have been accused of making arbitrary decisions that do nothing but impede research, almost for the sake of the impediment itself. Indeed, the *Policies and Procedures* manual for the University of Pennsylvania IRB (Version 1.0, October 24, 2001), on the first page, says, "the men and women who sit on Institutional Review Boards ... are ... expected to act as a gatekeeper, to slow down the drive of the research enterprise to find the newest therapy and to advance knowledge of the basics of biological and behavioral mechanisms." Because of the obstacles set up by IRBs, some potentially valuable research is not even attempted. In other cases, students suffer because of delays in approving their projects. Although each little revision and resubmission of the consent form may seem like a minor matter to those who require it, it becomes one more straw on the pile that researchers must already carry (which includes dealing with granting agencies and nasty journal reviewers), and these so-called minor concerns cost researchers months in delays. It may lead some to retire earlier than they would otherwise, to become dead wood, or to seek a different career. The "burden of red tape" is frequently cited as an obstacle to the economic development of poor countries (see, for example, Djankov et al. 2000), yet, in the field of research, it is ignored as trivial. Ultimately, it must have effects.

The burden is real. The staff of IRBs is growing, and the money must come from somewhere. Often the most harmless sort of study requires months of correspondence between researchers and IRB members to win approval. One such case was a series of studies in which I collaborated, with Peter Ubel of the University of Michigan and the Ann Arbor Veterans Affairs Medical Center. One study concerned the quality of life of patients undergoing kidney dialysis. We gave each patient a PDA (personal digital assistant), which beeped periodically. When the PDA beeped, the patient was supposed to answer a couple of questions about his mood. The idea was to measure aspects of the quality of life of patients that were not affected by biases of retrospection. An amendment to an already approved study was submitted to the IRB. It took nearly three months to obtain approval for modifications to recruiting procedures: permission to use a newspaper advertisement instead of recruiting only on campus, introduction of a prorated incentive payment to account for people who did not respond to the PDA during the week of their participation, minor changes to question wording, and related changes in the consent form. The IRB reviewer wanted to remove many questions from a questionnaire, some for the following reason: "Yes, these sections would give insight into how people view different 'health segments' within our society, but they do not in my opinion clearly follow from the PDA self evaluations the subjects have been doing." Obvious reply: So what? This reply was offered more politely in a lengthy e-mail message. The reviewer suggested many other changes, such as rewording questions, having nothing to do with risk to the subjects or whether they were informed. These were presented as requirements, not friendly suggestions. At one point, the review said of the single most important question in the study: "My personal recommendation would be to just drop this question." There was no evidence that the reviewer was an expert in the field of research in question. The reviewer also wanted the subjects paid in cash rather than checks, despite the risk to the researchers from carrying large amounts of cash. (The study did use cash, and no research assistant was injured.) The reviewer repeatedly insisted on telling the subjects that if the PDAs were lost they would not be replaced. Yet, this was not true.

For another research project that consisted of a series of questionnaires in a longitudinal study of patients' adaptation to spinal cord injury, it took eight and a half months to negotiate a series of surveys that satisfied the IRB. In another study, reviewers took issue with giving subjects candy as a token of appreciation for doing an anonymous survey; they were not satisfied with a "healthy snack" either and wanted to know what that would be. The researchers finally agreed to give out ballpoint pens instead. This concern, despite the fact that these same patients are offered free doughnuts in the same area. In another study, reviewers accused the researchers of deceiving subjects because, in an anonymous survey, they were not revealing their true hypothesis. Subjects were told, "We are interested in finding out how people think about life in different areas of the country"; in truth, the researchers were interested in the tendency of people to focus on what is different about having and not having a condition when they were evaluating it (the focusing illusion), and on the tendency to underpredict adaptation to the condition. One IRB administrator advised the researchers that they needed to get approval for *every* change to an anonymous survey *or* submit all the different possible versions for approval at the outset—even changing "a" to "the."

These interactions with IRBs occurred over the period of one year. Nobody I know who hears this story is surprised by it. Researchers have come to accept it. Lists of horror stories are easy to find. Here is one (from Sieber, Plattner, and Rubin 2002):

- An experimental economist seeking to do a laboratory-based study of betting choices in college seniors was held up for many months while their IRB considered and reconsidered the risks inherent in a study whose only real danger was boredom.

- A political scientist purchased appropriate names for a survey of voting behavior (of people who had consented to such participation) and was initially required by their IRB to get the written informed consent from subjects before mailing them the survey.

- A Caucasian Ph.D. student, seeking to study career expectations in relation to ethnicity, was told by the IRB that African-American PhD students could not be interviewed because it might be traumatic for them to be interviewed by the student.

- Faculty who employ routine classroom exercises for pedagogical purposes, in which students are asked to make judgments and discuss their reasons, are required by their IRBs to obtain the students' signed informed consent. The consent form includes the proviso that students may choose not to participate and warns of nonexistent risks. (No data are collected; no research is performed. The only purpose of the exercise is to educate the students.)

- Anonymity of subjects has been required for oral histories in which a single individual is interviewed about a historically significant event in which he or she was a key participant.

- A linguist seeking to study language development in a pre-literate tribe was instructed to have them read and sign a consent form.

IRBs successfully influence the attitudes of researchers, who often police each other and themselves. For example, a study by Chivers et al. (2004) was almost not done because the researchers' faculty colleagues thought that paying female subjects $75 to participate in a study of sexual arousal from watching sexually explicit videotapes—an idea designed to insure that the subjects were not doing it primarily because of interest in watching the tapes—was coercive (J. Michael Bailey, personal communication, Feb. 14, 2001; see section 8.1.1).

In sum, these IRBs have become like the Inquisition. They treat researchers as if they were potential heretics. They insist on purity of spirit, as evidenced through obsequious cooperation with their demands. They go well beyond their mandate to protect subjects, tinkering with every aspect of the research. There is also no evidence that they protect anyone from anything (Mueller and Fuerdy 2001).

The kind of research I do, once a joyful and harmless enterprise, has become a cause for shame, although it is still harmless. Perhaps it is indeed worthless. If so, then people should stop funding it, not kill it slowly with duck bites.

7.2.1   A proposal

The problem is what to do. A few points should be kept in mind when considering possible reform of the system.

- Researchers have a group interest in maintaining credibility. When public trust in the research enterprise declines, then researchers have trouble recruiting subjects.

- On the other hand, each individual researcher has an incentive to try to get a free ride on the trust placed in the enterprise as a whole, to try to get away with what he can. Putting this fact together with the last one, we can see that researchers have an incentive to police each other.

- Although IRBs have enormous power over researchers who are willing to go through the approval process, they have no way to discipline researchers who bypass the process or who renege on their promises after approval.

- The main incentive for researchers to go through the process is that granting agencies require it. Researchers who do not need grants can, and often do, skip the whole thing. The more difficult the approval process, the more this happens.

These points together imply a simple reform. The IRB should not require prior approval, at least not for innocuous categories of research. But its disciplinary power should increase. It should thus become more like committees that deal with scientific misconduct. Indeed, failure to inform subjects of risks and exaggeration of benefits are forms of scientific misconduct, potentially just as destructive to the enterprise of science as is plagiarism or the fudging of data. Researchers will not hesitate to punish such infractions.

One legal argument for such a reform is that IRBs prevent researchers from speaking freely to their subjects and others. In the United States, such censorship is arguably a violation of the First Amendment of the Constitution (Hamburger 2005). IRBs do this in subtle ways, by tinkering with the wording of questions, and also by intimidating researchers who might ask controversial or sensitive questions. Such researchers are often frightened away by the prospect of battles with the IRB.

Other relevant arguments come from the economic analysis of law. Shavell (2004, ch. 25), for example, considers the factors that should affect when law intervenes: before potential harmful acts are committed (e.g., through regulation), after the harmful acts but without waiting for harm (e.g., criminal sanctions against behavior that puts others at risk of harm), or after the harm occurs (e.g., tort law and contract law). Of course, the "law" here is a locally administered law, so the "state" is actually the IRB or its equivalent. My proposal is that the law should intervene at the point when risky behavior is committed, not before. The relevant factors fall into two categories, which concern information and sanctions, respectively.

7.2.2   Information held by the "state" vs. private parties

The issue here is who initiates legal action. Those in the best position to discover and report abuses are the subjects. The IRB, as it works now, uses prior regulation, and it faces severe limits on information. For one thing, it must rely completely on what investigators say. It has no way of detecting departures from stated protocols or omissions of relevant information about risks from the protocols. A far larger gap may be that many researchers do not submit protocols for approval at all. This occurs in areas of research that do not require grant support. The reputation of the IRB as slow and disorganized (at my institution) surely inhibits submissions that are not required in order to obtain funding. Moreover, even when proposals are submitted to the IRB, it must guess where the risks are from what the investigator says. IRBs do not generally inspect laboratories or send representatives to monitor research.

There are two problems with relying on subjects to report harm or risky behavior by researchers. One is that the subjects may lack information and make mistakes in both directions. The other is that some abuses involve taking advantage of a position of power over the subjects, and the same power will discourage subjects from reporting events.

Mistakes in which subjects report risks that are not really risks can be handled by investigation. The IRB will, under my proposal, investigate all such reports, typically by requiring the researcher to submit a protocol (i.e., what all researchers now must do) and to answer the allegations. More serious are cases in which the subject does not know the risk, for example, the risk of side effects of an experimental medication. Although the IRB may be able to detect such cases before the subject does, I suspect that most IRBs cannot do this either, unless researchers report the risks in their submissions to the IRB. If they voluntarily do this now, then they will probably inform their subjects too, under my proposal. I see no difference in the incentives placed on researchers to report risks truthfully as a function of whether the researcher deals directly with the subjects or first with the IRB.

The case of positions of power is a problem, but it is similar to the problem of sexual abuse of students and workers, for which we now rely on victims to report violations. The cases are different because of the extreme difficulty of using prior regulation to prevent sexual abuse. (Would it require, for example, that office doors be kept open during meetings between professors and students?) But there is a mechanism available for research that is not so easily available for sexual abuse— namely, giving "standing" to those who are not directly harmed. That is, people should be able to report risks even when they themselves are not subject to those risks. These people will include subjects but also anyone else, such as colleagues. Anonymous reports would be investigated.

7.2.3   Effectiveness and feasibility of sanctions

Prior regulation is most effective when sanctions are least effective. It is sometimes argued that we have no way to discipline researchers who break rules or cause harm. But, if this is true, we also have no way to discipline researchers who fail to do what they said they would do in the protocols they submitted, or who fail to submit complete protocols (or any protocols). And, in fact, discipline is possible, as illustrated in the Gelsinger case (chapter 1). Thus, ultimately, the system depends on both the honesty of researchers and the possibility of punishing them when they are caught. Arguably, a system that was less intrusive than the present system would increase honesty by placing trust in researchers (a mechanism supported by the findings of Bohnet, Frey, and Huck 2001).

There is at least one other major problem with this proposal (pointed out to me by David Laibson)—lawsuits. Universities, where most IRBs are, are "deep pockets" for lawsuits by subjects who are harmed in research. Current law in the United States would not permit a university to pass this buck to the researcher, and, even if it could, the possibility of doing so would deter many people from research careers. Thus, universities have a strong interest in protecting themselves from lawsuits, and the threat of discipline may not be enough to induce a researcher to take sufficient care. The university's interest is greater than the researcher's because the university has more to lose. Because of the university's interest, it may reasonably require prior approval of certain classes of research, specifically those that might lead to lawsuits.

Two factors, however, suggest that prior approval will not have much benefit in reducing lawsuits: the unpredictability of the legal system and the unpredictability of adverse outcomes.

Unpredictability of the law

When adverse outcomes happen, the victims of them often look for someone to sue, especially in the United States (which, arguably, has substituted a plaintiff-friendly legal system for a generous social safety net). I have already discussed some of the problems of tort law in section 6.8. Another problem is unpredictability.

Studies of medical malpractice have found that most cases of negligent behavior do not lead to lawsuits, that winning a lawsuit is much more closely tied to the magnitude of the injury than to the extent of malpractice, and that lawsuits do not seem to deter negligent behavior (Brennan, Sox, and Burstin 1996; Kessler and McClellan 2002; Localio et al. 1991). Changes in the rules to make it harder for plaintiffs to win large sums of money have no detectable effect on injuries.

Part of the problem seems to be that the legal system is so unpredictable. Doctors practice "defensive medicine"—that is, perform tests and procedures because they think they could get sued for not performing them, even though these may not be in the best interest of the patient (DeKay and Asch 1998). Doctors who lose lawsuits often do not think they did anything wrong. In this case, they are unlikely to change their behavior in ways that would be better for patients.

The tort system in medicine, and probably elsewhere, has become something of a wild card. Getting sued is a random, unpredictable event, like getting caught in a traffic jam on an interstate highway.

If there is an incentive effect, it is more to discourage people from occupations that get sued a lot, such as obstetrics. People are particularly likely to sue when the injury is done to a healthy person, or a person expected to be healthy. Oncologists who do cancer therapy are rarely sued for its side effects.

It is not surprising that the law is so unpredictable. Judgments of all sorts are unpredictable, including those of boards such as IRBs (Plous and Herzog 2001).

Prediction of adverse outcomes

There are two kinds of adverse outcomes that an IRB must try to predict. The first is simply harm to the subject. The second is harm that might lead to a successful lawsuit. Presumably, the second category is included within the first, but even that cannot be assumed. People sue for harms not caused by those they sue (e.g., spontaneously arising illnesses) and win. The most important component of the second category is what IRBs spend most of their time worrying about: harms not anticipated in the consent form that the subject has read. Of course, prediction of unanticipated harms requires prediction of harms.

Researchers have an interest in downplaying such possibilities, but they have more information than IRBs. Can IRBs improve the situation?

IRBs often try to anticipate low-probability events. When reviewing a study involving functional magnetic resonance imaging (fMRI), the panel I was on spent several minutes discussing the possibility that subjects would neglect instructions to remove metal objects. Because fMRI involves a powerful magnet, metal objects can fly at high speeds and cause serious injury or death. The problem was whether the consent form should list all the various sorts of objects that subjects might not think of.

How good are people at predicting such low-probability events? If I answered, "not very good," you would want to know just what that means. Compared to what? And what counts as "good?" A better answer will require some mathematical reasoning and a few assumptions. The conclusion we can draw is that errors increase as probability decreases. Thus, the capacity to predict very low-probability events is poor compared to that for predicting higher-probability events.

First, let us assume that the tendency to worry about low probability events increases in proportion to the seriousness of the consequence. Death from a flying metal object is a very serious consequence, so it is worth thinking about low-probability events that might lead to it. As a rough approximation, it seems worth assuming that the concern will depend on the expected disutility, ED, of the event. Thus, the seriousness of what people worry about, its ED, will not depend on probability. As probability decreases, disutility increases proportionally, so that the overall ED is about the same.

Second, let us assume that there is an ED threshold (EDT) for including an item in a warning or consent form. The threshold could be calculated to minimize the losses resulting from both possible errors: failing to warn about a real risk and warning unnecessarily. The latter error is costly because it dilutes attention. The more risks we warn about, the less attention people will pay to each warning, and the less likely they are to act on it. Thus, there is a loss for either error. The expected loss depends on the distance from the threshold. If the ED is very close to the EDT, then the expected cost of the misclassification will be low.

Third, suppose that the judges, the IRB, proceed as if they made probability judgments for each risk. The errors will be greater and more likely when the variability in these judgments is greater.

Fourth, the seriousness of the errors will depend only on their size— expressed as a ratio between ED and EDT—not on the probability of the bad event. This assumption follows from the first assumption.

Given these assumptions, we can estimate the seriousness of errors by looking at the variability of probability on a logarithmic scale. The use of a logarithmic scale insures that a given ratio of error expresses itself as a constant difference. For example, if the threshold for a given bad event is reached when the probability is .01, an omission error based on a probability judgment of .001 would represent a ratio of 1/10. This error would, I assume, be just as bad in a case when the threshold is .001 and the probability judgment is .0001—the same ratio. This is because, by the first assumption, the disutility of the bad event is 10 times as great when the threshold is .001 than when the threshold is .01.

To estimate how variability depends on probability, I used a data set in which we asked two groups of subjects to make judgments of the probability of various bad events on a logarithmic scale (Baron, Hershey, and Kunreuther 2000). The bad events ranged from "injury or death from an asteroid hitting the earth" to "bacterial infection from contaminated food." The former is, of course, extremely unlikely yet absolutely awful, while the latter is fairly likely to occur to most people and, on the average, not very serious. One group of subjects, the experts, consisted of 122 members of the Society for Risk Analysis who returned a mail questionnaire. The other group consisted of 150 nonexperts who completed the study on the World Wide Web.

For each bad event, and for each group, I computed the standard deviation (s.d.) of the (base 10) log probability judgments across subjects. Figure 7.2 shows the results. Each point is a particular bad event. It is apparent that, for both groups, the lower the probability, the higher the variability of the judgments. Across the 32 events, the correlation between log probability and its s.d. was statistically significant for each group ($r = -.54$, $p = .0013$, for experts; $r = -.63$, $p = .0001$, for nonexperts). In sum, the lower the probability, the greater the expected error.[2]

What is to be done about this situation is not obvious. We cannot just say "give up" when the probabilities become low. It is reasonable to assume, as I have assumed, that we don't even worry about very low-probability events unless they are very bad. We should and do worry, for instance, about the threat posed by asteroids, despite the low probability.

Perhaps one thing we can do is to distribute our effort where it would do the most good. Probability judgments can presumably be improved by combining the judgments of several judges. That takes more time, and we would want to do it when it would do the most good, specifically, for low-probability events. The judgments are also surely more accurate if they are made by those who know the most.

But IRBs as they are currently constituted do not do this. They spend a few minutes imagining scenarios, and then insist on a revision of the consent form. Researchers are in a better position to analyze the risks. They know more and have more time.

On the other hand, despite the fact that prior IRB approval is unlikely to reduce harm in a predictable way, it may still provide a defense in court. The very unpredictability of the system suggests that it attends to

---

[2]The point at the far left would have a higher s.d., but responses below 10^{-10} were raised to 10^{-10}. This was, of course, the asteroid.

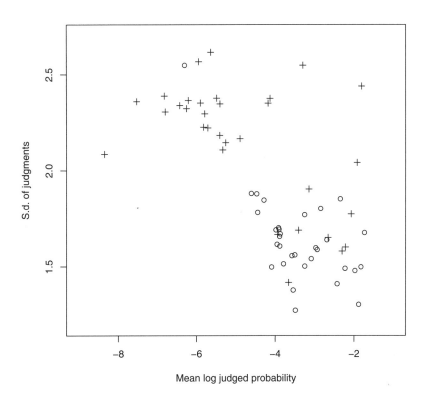

Figure 7.2: Standard deviation of log probability judgments as a function of their mean (experts, +; nonexperts, ○)

irrelevant factors and ignores relevant ones. Prior approval may still be helpful for some categories of research, such as those in which physical injury is an inherent risk.

7.3   Privacy

Researchers often ask for confidential data about their subjects, sometimes even without subjects' permission.

7.3.1   Privacy as a means value

In general, privacy is a means value (as defined in section 3.4). That is, we value privacy because we could be harmed by the use or misuse of personal information about us. We could be denied insurance on the basis of medical information, and this is harmful even if the information is correct. Our money could be stolen if someone gets our credit card number. We could be embarrassed if someone finds out what Web sites we've been looking at, or fired if an employer finds out.

The case of embarrassment is interesting because it might seem that embarrassment is inseparable from privacy violation, so privacy is not a means to avoid embarrassment, as I have claimed. Instead, it could be that violation of privacy about certain matters is exactly what is embarrassing. I do not think so, though. Rather, it seems to me that what is embarrassing is knowing that someone knows that you look at pictures of naked ladies. It's not embarrassing for me to know that someone knows that I regularly read Slashdot and the Yahoo finance page. (See. I just told you.)

Of course, if you broke into my computer and discovered that I read Slashdot, then I might be angry. Why? Could it be that I have a fundamental value for privacy, or is this still a means value? In the next section, I discuss how privacy might become a fundamental value, but I don't think this is an example of it. I think this is just anger at someone breaking the law, or a convention that has the force of law.

7.3.2   Privacy and trust

Consider a medical research study that will collect information about many patients, without their knowledge or consent. You are in charge of approving that study. You know, with 100 percent certainty, that the information will be used for research purposes only. It will not be released to anyone, and the researchers will not know the patients' names, so the patients will not suffer any embarrassment through revelations to the researchers. The research itself will be beneficial, if it succeeds. In sum, no harm can come from this research, at least no harm of the usual sort, and some benefit is possible.

This is roughly what happened in a controversial case in Iceland (Merz, McGee, and Sankar 2004; Hoeyer and Lynöe 2004). The case was complicated by the involvement of a private company, which stood to profit from the data. Most of the dispute hinges on legal and legalistic interpretations of documents such as the Declaration of Helsinki. I do not want to discuss this case, but rather a general issue that it raises in connection with means values.

People may be opposed to allowing their own data to be used not only because they believe they might be harmed but also because they disapprove of the general purpose of the research and wish to discourage it. Both concerns are about trust. They must trust the researchers not only to protect them from harm but also to do something useful with the data. The desire to withhold data could result from a belief that one of these conditions is not met. Because the desire is based on a belief, it is a means value. When a private company is using the data, the general-purpose trust issue may come to the fore, because people may be more likely to think that the company will use the data for private profit rather than public good.

The idea of withholding data because of disapproval of the apparent general purpose amounts to a kind of political judgment rather than a personal protection. Withholding data is a way of voting against the research. Indeed, the more people who do this, the more the research suffers as a result. It would be just as much of a vote against the proposal if anyone else's data were withheld.

In many situations, governments have the power to compel cooperation with a project, for example, the military draft or taxes. Presumably, the same issues of mistrust arise in these cases. Surely, though, this is a legitimate function of government. In a democracy, if the government pushes too hard against public mistrust, it loses support.

7.3.3 Expectation and incentive

Protection of privacy has costs. Medical costs could be reduced, and errors avoided, if medical records were more easily shared. Research could proceed more efficiently if researchers could gain access to patients' records without permission. Clinical psychologists could prevent harm by sharing what they learn with police or with those endangered by their clients. Suppose that we allowed such privacy invasions?

Three things would happen. First, we would get the benefits. Second, harmful invasions of privacy would increase. In each case, the balance of these two effects is relevant to decisions about the appropriate level of privacy protection. The third effect is that people would, over time, adjust their behavior to the new rules. This adjustment, itself, would have costs and benefits.

For example, if psychologists' clients learned that the psychologists could share information with police or relatives, they would watch what they said. They would not admit to wanting to harm someone, or even perhaps to wanting to kill themselves. In this case, reduced privacy protection might do more harm than good.

In some cases, the adjustments might be short lived. For example, if restrictions on researchers' access to patient data were eased, some people might initially be more reluctant to volunteer for research studies, or even to seek medical treatment, for fear that their complaint would be discovered. (For example, people who wanted a high-level security clearance might be more reluctant to seek psychotherapy.) But if the researchers almost never violate privacy in harmful ways, these mistrusting adjustments will eventually stop.

In other cases, the adjustments might not be so harmful because they might simply involve taking more care, *caveat emptor*. Most people have become a little wary about giving their credit card numbers on the Internet. They demand some evidence of trustworthiness in order to do it. The same might happen for participation in research. Indeed, even now, "rogue research," done outside of the purview of any review body, is done by telephone interviewers who pose as consumer surveyors but are actually trying to sell a product. When people are contacted by a legitimate research interviewer, they become wary and ask a few questions before proceeding. This is not a great cost.

7.3.4   What if privacy becomes fundamental?

Harm can result from a research study if some of the patients value their privacy for its own sake. Even though they do not know that their privacy is being violated, this violation goes against something they value. The lack of knowledge is irrelevant. We have values that we want honored, even when we do not know about violations, so we should endorse rules that respect them. Privacy may have started out as a means value, but now it is a fundamental value, valued independently of whether it is a means to other ends (see section 3.4).

Although we must honor such a value in privacy for its own sake, we must recognize it as an "evil desire"—namely, a value that conflicts with the values of others. If it is allowed to win, in this case, the research will be prevented or hampered, and the expected benefits of the research will be reduced. The additional utility that results from discouraging such desires might be sufficient to override them, even when they would otherwise tilt the balance toward their side. Or it might not.

What is the difference between such an evil desire and a simple self-interested desire? Most self-interested values also conflict with the values of others. If one person eats more, then less is available for others. I suggest that there are two differences.

First, self-interested desires are not very malleable. It does little good to try to discourage them, since discouragement will have little effect. Hunger is very basic.

Second, and more important, the simple, basic self-interested desires are desired themselves. Despite the claims of Buddhism that desires are "attachments" that are best gotten rid of, the basic desires are things that most of us would rather have than not have, even given the fact that they are not always satisfied. (Consider a pill to rid people of sexual desire, to be taken by those who know that their desires would not be satisfied. Most people would not want such a pill, I suspect.)

We would not want a desire for privacy if it were not a means to other things that we want. It causes only pain and worry. There is no pleasure in knowing that our privacy is protected. Thus, we have another reason to discourage such values: they are bad for the people who hold them. This is not true of most basic self-interested values. Nor is it true even of labile self-interested values, such as appreciation of artistic expression.

7.4   Conclusion

I have argued that potential conflict of interest between researchers and subjects are often less than meet the eye. These are, of course, one example of conflict of interest. Others are between physicians and patients, or insurers and patients. What an insurer calls "insurance fraud" may be, in the eyes of a physician, an honest attempt to remedy an unjust decision about coverage.

I have focused here on the widely felt problem of the intrusiveness of IRBs. I have proposed a solution, in which the amount of prior review of research is cut back in favor of clear guidelines and a punishment mechanism for violations. A reviewer of an earlier version of this section argued, "The protections of human subjects have been instituted because violations have previously occurred, just as traffic lights are installed at intersections with high accident rates. This restriction on movement applies to all drivers, not only those who have had accidents at that intersection, and seems to be a reasonable price to pay for public safety." Let us follow this analogy. Traffic lights are exactly what I am proposing, in the form of clear guidelines. What happens now is that, before I go for a drive, I must submit my itinerary for approval, promising that I will look both ways at every intersection. What is missing now are the red lights. If we had them, and if I had to pass a drivers test on the rules, I would not need to go through this approval process before each trip.

More generally, attempts to regulate conflict of interest must consider the actual consequences of increased regulation. When people are mistrusted, they become less trustworthy. If they are incompletely monitored, they may perform worse than if they were simply trusted from the outset. Violations will, of course, still occur, as they do everywhere in life, but they can be dealt with after the fact, as crimes are.

Chapter 8

Drug Research

According to Frank Lichtenberg (2002; see also Lichtenberg 2004), expenditures on drug research and development between 1960 and 1997 in the United States were a major determinant of the increase in life expectancy from 69.7 to 76.5 years. In particular, the expenditure of $1,345 on research and development increased one person's life expectancy by a year. Even if this figure is a substantial underestimate of the cost, it seems likely that drug research is one of the more efficient ways to improve health and prolong life. Of course, if more money were spent, the benefits per dollar would decline. So the real import of Lichtenberg's result is that more money could be spent efficiently on drug research, up to some level that is surely higher than present expenditures.

Moreover, the process of approving new drugs is slow, and the delay actually causes harm (Bazerman, Baron, and Shonk 2001; Rubin 2005). Arguably, both public policy and individual decisions by officials are influenced by a decision-making bias in which harms of omission tend to be ignored (as I discuss in section 9.1.1).

8.1   Recruiting subjects for drug trials

One way to spend money might be to speed up drug trials. Some trials fail because they never recruit the required number of subjects. Others take much longer than they could (Alger 1999). Yet, only 3 percent of cancer patients participate in trials, and the number of patients in the typical phase III trial—the final phase before approval—is increasing, making the trials take longer. It is now over 4,000 subjects for the average trial (Alger 1999). Can we improve the recruitment of subjects? (In section 8.2.2, I shall suggest how we might reduce the need for them with better statistical procedures.) Cancer drugs require an average of four years for phase III trials, sometimes much longer. Some of these drugs will turn out to be effective. Lives are thus being lost because of these delays. We don't know whose lives, of course, because we don't know which drugs are successful, and which patients would be saved by them.

8.1.1   Paying subjects: Coercion? Undue influence?

The ethical rules for drug trials are a complex mixture of law, regulation, and custom. Many are administered through IRBs of universities and other research institutions that receive United States government research funds. Institutions that receive these funds must have an IRB, and most drug research still involves these institutions.

IRBs typically meet once or twice a month and review dozens of proposals in a meeting of two or three hours. Each proposal is a few pages. It includes a summary of the research plan and a sample consent form that the subject is supposed to read and sign. Of course, a couple of members of the panel, at least, have read each proposal beforehand. IRBs are composed of a mix of people—doctors and nurses who work with patients, doctors and nurses who do research, other researchers, clergymen, lawyers, and interested patients. They must make sure that the subjects are well informed about the experiments they are to enter and that the subjects are not coerced, and do not feel coerced. They are also supposed to make sure that the potential benefits of the research outweigh the risks; in fact, though, the mix of people involved in IRBs makes them unqualified to evaluate the scientific quality of research proposals.

Many members of IRBs feel that payment is a form of coercion (see chapter 6). Studies that pay too much are generally sent back for revision. That can cause delay for another month. Researchers do not wait to be told this. They have heard that this happens, and they typically censor themselves. If any of them are tempted to increase their rate of enrolling subjects by paying more, they suppress the temptation.

However, higher pay might benefit everyone. The drug companies and even the government may be willing to pay more to increase the rate of subject enrollment. The drug companies are concerned about profits, of course, especially when the patent's life begins at the time when testing begins, not at the time a drug is approved. Only with a patent can a company profit from having a monopoly on the drug. But patients in need of the drugs also benefit from faster approval.

What about the subjects? Two arguments are made about why they should not be paid too much. One is that it takes away their choice. If you make the pay high enough, almost everyone will accept it. If everyone accepts it, then their behavior is determined so that they have no free will. Hence, they have lost their choice. This is nonsense. The point of the idea of autonomy is that people should be able to choose what is best for them according to their own values. If people value money so much that sufficient amounts of money will induce them to do something, that is one of their values. They think they are better off taking the money. Unless we have good reason to think they are wrong, we should take their word for it. They think they are better off with the money, and it is very likely that they are. So, if the subjects are better off, if the companies and their stockholders are better off, and if future patients are better off, this is a win-win-win proposition.

This simple-minded confusion of autonomy and unpredictability is not the only problem, though. There are real concerns that money will induce subjects to make decisions that they would later regret according to their own values. They might, for example, skim over the section of the consent form dealing with "potentially dangerous side effects" for fear that they might discover something that would scare them away. And perhaps they should sometimes be scared away despite the money.

Still, this concern is always there whatever the subject's reason for participating in a study. Even if a patient is participating out of sheer altruism, the strong desire to help others with the same disease might cause her to skim over the risks in just the same way. The solution to the problem—and there is no evidence that it is a problem—is to try harder to make sure that the subject is aware of the risks. (Later, I suggest an experimental approach to this issue.)

The idea of protecting autonomy extends further than money. Most consent forms do not include any information at all about the potential benefits of the research to others. Yet, that is the best of all reasons to participate in research, altruism (see section 6.6). IRBs tend to think that mentioning these benefits will induce guilt feelings in those who decline to participate. The upshot of this is to make the consent form almost useless as an aid to the real decision. The subject must simply guess about the benefits to others. Many subjects who do participate have faith in the progress of science that perhaps should not extend to the particular study in which they are participating.

Although high payments to subjects are strongly discouraged, high payments to doctors have recently become a small scandal. Patients get into drug studies mostly because their own doctors suggest it to them. The doctors are often involved in the study as researchers. Sometimes, though, they play little active part in the design or analysis of the research. Their main role is to recruit patients for the study. If they really think this benefits their own patients, they might do this because they see it as part of being a good doctor. Often this happens. But often, too, the benefits of the research itself will accrue mostly to others. Before a drug is approved, it is not clear yet whether it is good for the patient. It might even be bad.

IRBs do not generally frown upon the idea of paying doctors small amounts of money "for expenses" in recruiting patients for drug studies. Recently, though, the need for subjects has led to some examples of very high payments (Eichenwald and Kolata, *New York Times*, May 16, 1999; Lemmens and Miller 2003). Typically, this happens when drug companies hire other companies to do the actual testing. These contractors are not so bound by fear of losing their good reputations as are the companies that employ them. (But sometimes the big companies do it too.) They offer hundreds of dollars for each patient who is signed up for a clinical trial. "Expenses" could not possibly justify this. Some doctors have made over $100,000 in a year just from recruiting subjects. Much of this research, since it is privately funded and done by private contractors, is unsupervised by any IRB.

The ethical problems here seem more real to us than those of paying patients. Patients have the strong incentive of looking out for their own interest. If they decide that the money makes up for the risk of side effects, and if they are truly informed, then we have little reason to question this judgment. Doctors usually try to be advocates for their patients' interests. But the offer of large amounts of money to doctors puts them in a different kind of conflict. The conflict for patients is between two of their own interests, avoiding risk and making money. The conflict for doctors is between their own interests and their patients' interests. Pay them enough, and they will look hard for reasons why they really ought to recommend drug trial X to patient Y, despite the fact that Y doesn't clearly have the disease in question and is at possible risk for some of the anticipated side effects of the drug.

The irony is that this problem would not have arisen if patients themselves could be paid. We are facing an amazing situation in which doctors are paid to enroll patients when the patients themselves cannot be paid because it is "unethical." The idea of trading money for risk is seen as an ethical violation.

Grady (2001) reviews the United States rules prohibiting "coercion or undue influence." She argues that payments are not coercion, because coercion is a threat of harm. One might argue about the distinction between causing harm and failing to provide a benefit. From a utilitarian perspective (which Grady does not take), one might argue that it is a net harm if a subject participates only to avoid a consequence that is worse than if the study were not available at all. If the subject is rational, then this is a sign that the study itself is harmful to him. (The harm might still be outweighed by benefits to others.) Thus, the offer of payment cannot be harmful in this sense, unless the payment would be due anyway if the study were not available. (See also chapter 6.)

A bigger question is whether large payments could amount to undue influence, whether they are "excessively influential," or whether they are "inappropriate" (the term used in the Belmont Report). What could these terms mean? One possibility is that, as Grady puts it (p. 42): "Money certainly has a reputation for getting people to do things they otherwise would not do, and, in some cases, for getting people to do something they know is wrong. Hence, we see daily newspaper accounts of scandals, bribes, and extortion. Money is also believed capable of inappropriately distorting people's judgments and motivations." Money could blind people to risks, or cause them to lie about risk factors that could exclude them from the study, thus putting themselves at greater risk.

The latter case is arguably a problem of information. Suppose the experimenter said, "If you have a heart condition, this experiment has a

50 percent chance of killing you." Then a subject who knowingly participated with a heart condition would be making a decision with the relevant information at hand. Perhaps the issue here is whether such a decision would itself be a sign of incompetence to consent (as discussed in section 6.7).

But could money blind people to risks? Casarett, Karlawish, and Asch (2002) found that many potential subjects—jurors in Philadelphia—thought that very high payments might impair other people's ability to think carefully about the risks and benefits of a clinical trial. Very few thought that payment would impair their own judgment.

Whether money distorts judgment is an empirical question, but we have no reason to think that it would. Here is the kind of experiment required to do the empirical test. We would ask subjects to consent to a series of research studies. We look for what factors put them right on the borderline between consenting and not consenting. (We might use a numerical judgment scale, in which the middle point indicates exact indifference.) The subject might be told that one of them is real and that their answer to this study will determine whether they are asked to join it. (If the subject is indifferent, a coin is flipped.) The items in the series will vary in at least three dimensions: money; a risk dimension, such as probability of a serious side effect; and a second benefit dimension, more "legitimate" than money, such as the chance for a cure of a condition they have.[1] If money blinds people to risks, then the higher the value of the money dimension, the less people will attend to the risk dimension. We can estimate their attention to the risk by asking how it trades off with the second benefit. How much of the second benefit is required to compensate for a given increase in the risk? (That is, if both the risk and the benefit increase and the judgment stays the same, then we can say that the increase in benefit compensates for the increase in risk.) Thus, the hypothesis predicts that less of the second benefit is needed to compensate for a given increase in risk as the amount of money increases.

If this result is not found, we may still find that money affects the judgment. But that is not the problem. It is rational to want more money.

---

[1]Note that the second benefit must be considered as a legitimate inducement. If no inducement is legitimate, then we are back to the situation in which the only reasons for subjects to consent are that they are irrational or that they do not believe what they are told.

The claim is rather that money distorts the judgment of other factors. I know of no psychological mechanism that could explain the result, even if it were found.

Another reason why paying subjects too much might be wrong is that it amounts to a kind of prostitution, or "commodification" of what should not be sold.[2] If you accept a large amount of money to put yourself at risk, you are selling your body. The same issue is raised in a more pointed way about other kinds of sales, such as sales of organs, and I shall therefore discuss it further in section 9.2.2.

Payment is not the only form of coercion that apparently confuses IRBs. Daniel Wikler (personal communication, Oct. 10, 2003) provided the following account of an IRB's attitude:

> In a study of HIV mother-to-child transmission in Africa, in-vestigators wanted to approach women about to give birth to ask if they planned to breast-feed. If the answer was yes, they'd invite the woman to be in their study, and they made participation attractive by guaranteeing two years of antiret-roviral treatment, plus an effort to secure more. The commit-tee didn't object to the antiretroviral offer—it's now standard to *require* that, to fulfill the "best available treatment" clause of the Declaration of Helsinki), but they were forbidden to mention it to women until after they'd answered the ques-tion about whether they intended to breastfeed. Reason: this would coerce them into breastfeeding, and thus deny them their autonomy.

The researchers may have wanted to avoid subjects who said they would breast-feed, and then did not follow through. But this was not the concern of the IRB. Rather, they thought that anything that might swing the decision about breast feeding must be coercive. Anything that affects someone's decision is a violation of autonomy (even if many other factors, such as family advice, have already affected it).

---

[2]This was suggested to me by John Sabini.

8.1.2   Using subjects in poor countries: Exploitation?

Another way of getting subjects is to do the studies in poor countries. This has two advantages for drug developers. First, if the subjects are to be paid in any form, the pay goes much farther. Sometimes it is considered legitimate, even in the United States, to provide some free medical care in return for participation in a study. For most people in the United States, this is not a big incentive because their medical care is mostly paid for anyway by private or government insurance. But most Africans, for example, have had very little, if any, of what people in rich countries call medical care. This can be a very strong incentive.

Many have objected that use of subjects in poor countries amounts to exploitation, and, on this ground, they want to prohibit, or strictly limit, research using poor subjects in poor countries. What could exploitation be that makes it wrong? One possibility is that exploitation is a form of coercion. This does not seem to be the problem with using poor people as subjects. They are not threatened with the loss of anything that they would get otherwise in the absence of the offer to participate.

Another possibility is that the researchers are taking advantage of a bad situation. This is, of course, true. The researchers benefit by having to pay less than they would pay in their own countries, and they would not be able to do this if income were equally distributed around the world. But are they making the situation worse than by not doing the study at all, or by doing it in their home countries? It is difficult to argue that they are making the situation worse than these two alternatives. In the case of not doing the study at all—and sometimes this is the main alternative—the poor subjects would do without income that they would otherwise get, and future patients, wherever they might be, would lose the benefits of the research. As for the alternative of doing the study at home, this would cost more, thus limiting future research or the scope of the present research. And people in poor countries presumably need the money more than those who would participate in rich countries. Because they live in such poverty, they have fewer ways to make money at all. At the very least, we have no reason to think the reverse—namely, that the subjects in rich countries need the money more.

The idea of exploitation might come down to a sense of unfairness, in two respects. First, the subjects in the poor countries might be getting less than the researchers are in fact able to pay. If, for example, they were to bargain collectively with the researchers, they might get more than they were initially offered. The same would not be true if the subjects came from a rich country, since the researchers would already (we assume) be stretched to the limit of what they could pay; they could not easily ask a funding agency for more funds for the purpose of giving more pay to their subjects than the going rate. From a utilitarian perspective, the behavior of the researchers in this case—in which they could pay more but do not—is still better than not doing the study at all or doing it in a rich country, but perhaps not as good as possible.

The issue is the long-term trade-off between spending more money now and saving money for future research. If researchers all started saying, "I want to do this study in central Africa, but I will pay the U.S. rate," they would not save money for granting agencies and companies that sponsor their research. It may be that saving money would lead to more beneficial research, which would provide greater long-term benefits than giving the money to subjects now. Or it may not.[3] In any case, this seems to be the empirical question at issue. Although it may seem like a good idea to ask researchers to help the world's poor by doing more for their subjects, one could also argue that researchers are no better situated than anyone else in rich countries to be asked to help the poor. For example, rich countries could raise taxes and increase foreign aid for health services—or anything.

A second source of the sense of unfairness is the possibility that the subjects are drawn from some group that will not benefit from the research as much as some other group. The subjects are being paid to take risks for someone else. Of course, this is usually true to some extent: many experiments fail yet are part of the whole enterprise that leads to benefits, and, even when treatments are beneficial, researchers may learn over time how to reduce their risks.

But, consider the most extreme case, in which people in poor countries are given a drug that they will be unable to afford once it is developed. (Again, let us admit that it is a bad thing that they cannot afford the drug and a good thing to correct this situation in any way.) If they

---

[3]Note that this strategy of paying poor people at a much higher rate runs into the usual questions about coercion with money, but of course I have argued against that concern.

want the money enough to take the risk, and if they are adequately informed and rational in pursuing their own self-interest, then the study would benefit them, not harm them. The situation is much the same as the case of not paying them enough: there are better options, perhaps even better options for the researchers, but this is not by itself sufficient reason to reject a study when it is the only option on the table.

8.2   Placebo controls

A real case concerns some experiments done in Africa to test new therapies for AIDS. In 1994, Connor et al. reported that zidovudine (AZT) reduced the rate of transmission of HIV (human immunodeficiency virus, the cause of AIDS) from mother to newborn by over 50 percent, in the United States and France. Soon after the results were known, several other studies began in poor countries (Lurie and Wolfe 1997). The experiments were initiated because most pregnant African women with AIDS cannot afford the usual treatment—a complex sequence of administrations of the drug AZT—given to prevent their children from catching the disease. The experiments involved comparing new drugs and shorter courses of AZT within a control group. The problem was that the control group was to be given only a placebo, an inactive drug. A no-treatment control is the fastest way to learn whether the new treatment is effective. (The placebo reduces the psychological effects of knowing whether one is getting treatment or not.) In the United States, it is typical not to use placebo controls in such studies, but rather to use the best available alternative treatment. However, the best available alternative treatment in Africa is no treatment at all. Moreover, it would be pointless to compare the newer treatments to the usual form of AZT treatment given in the United States, since the new treatment would very likely be somewhat less effective, and the standard treatment could not be used in Africa because of its cost. If the new treatment were found to be a little less effective than the standard treatment, it would still be nearly impossible to tell whether it was sufficiently better than nothing, without a placebo control group.

Arguably then, the choice was between giving the treatment to half the subjects or to none at all. Still, Public Citizen, a consumer-advocacy organization in the United States (headed by Ralph Nader), protested the trials because they were "unethical," and some members of Congress agreed (Cohen 1997). So did the editor of the *New England Journal of Medicine*, who wrote an editorial about the general problem (Angell 1997), which was followed by other comments on both sides (for example, Lurie and Wolfe 1997, who were at the time the heads of Public Citizen's Health Research Group; Varmus and Satcher 1997). Rothman (2000) provides a good and balanced summary account from the perspective of those opposed to the trials.

This is a clear case of a moral intuition about fairness getting in the way of people's good. No good at all would result from canceling the experiment. But the experiment itself could save the lives of many children, and it could lead to knowledge that would save the lives of many more.

The first paragraph of Angell (1997) lays out the position against the trials (citations deleted):

> An essential ethical condition for a randomized clinical trial comparing two treatments for a disease is that there be no good reason for thinking one is better than the other. Usually, investigators hope and even expect that the new treatment will be better, but there should not be solid evidence one way or the other. If there is, not only would the trial be scientifically redundant, but the investigators would be guilty of knowingly giving inferior treatment to some participants in the trial. The necessity for investigators to be in this state of equipoise applies to placebo-controlled trials, as well. Only when there is no known effective treatment is it ethical to compare a potential new treatment with a placebo. When effective treatment exists, a placebo may not be used. Instead, subjects in the control group of the study must receive the best known treatment. Investigators are responsible for all subjects enrolled in a trial, not just some of them, and the goals of the research are always secondary to the well-being of the participants. Those requirements are made clear in the Declaration of Helsinki of the World Health

Organization (WHO), which is widely regarded as providing the fundamental guiding principles of research involving human subjects. It states, "In research on man [sic], the interest of science and society should never take precedence over considerations related to the wellbeing of the subject," and "In any medical study, every patient—including those of a control group, if any—should be assured of the best proven diagnostic and therapeutic method."

From a decision-theoretic perspective, this doesn't make much sense. First, complete equipoise is, to say the least, rare. For perfect equipoise, the EU of the two treatments would have to be equal. But researchers can almost always find some reason to think that one treatment would have higher EU. Given that treatments almost always differ in EU, what counts as a big enough difference?

Second, if we put the interests of subjects first, that means that we never reduce the EU of any subject in order to gain knowledge that will help others. If we took this literally, we would almost never do any research. If we did not take it literally, where do we draw the line?

A third issue, of course, is what are the other options? If Angell's guidelines were taken literally, the research would not get done. There was no option to give the control group a treatment that was simply unaffordable. Decision theory compares options to other real options. Ethics seems to compare some options to something else, and then, finding them deficient, rejects them. I shall return to this issue.

A decision-theoretic analysis can point to real costs of hurting subjects in order to help others. The main cost, after the harm itself, is loss of trust in research. If subjects thought that the overall EU of entering an experiment was less than refusing, they would refuse. If they think that experimenters lie about the risks, then they would be even more inclined to refuse. This would make it more difficult for researchers to recruit subjects in the future, and that, in turn, would reduce the potential gains from research. But this was not an issue in the study in question. The control subjects got almost nothing, but they were still better off than if they had not participated at all, and each subject had a chance of being in the active condition.

8.2.1   Statistical issues

Angell (1997) does make one argument that requires serious consideration here, namely, that the use of placebo controlled trials might be excessive because of "slavish adherence to the tenets of clinical trials," which, presumably, demand placebo controls if at all possible.

Varmus and Satcher (1997; see also the correspondence in *New England Journal of Medicine, 338*, number 12), argue:

> For example, testing two or more interventions of unknown benefit (as some people have suggested) will not necessarily reveal whether either is better than nothing. Even if one surpasses the other, it may be difficult to judge the extent of the benefit conferred, since the interventions may differ markedly in other ways – for example, cost or toxicity. A placebo-controlled study would supply that answer. Similarly, comparing an intervention of unknown benefit – especially one that is affordable in a developing country – with the only intervention with a known benefit (the 076 regimen) may provide information that is not useful for patients. If the affordable intervention is less effective than the 076 regimen – not an unlikely outcome – this information will be of little use in a country where the more effective regimen is unavailable. Equally important, it will still be unclear whether the affordable intervention is better than nothing and worth the investment of scarce health care dollars.

On the other side, Lurie and Wolfe (1997) argued, "We believe that such equivalency studies of alternative antiretroviral regimens [as were being conducted in Thailand] will provide even more useful results than placebo-controlled trials." Lurie and Wolfe go on to argue that equivalence studies are not significantly slower, and that about the same number of subjects are required for meaningful results.

The traditional statistical approach relies on null-hypothesis testing. The idea is to compare two conditions—such as drug vs. placebo or new drug vs. old drug. The question is whether the two conditions differ. The data consist of numbers from the experimental condition, such as number of babies with HIV, and corresponding numbers from the control condition. For example, with 100 subjects in each condition, 60 might have HIV in the control condition and 30 in the experimental (drug) condition. The question is whether the conditions differ or, alternatively, whether the apparent difference is just chance. To test this, we make the assumption that the conditions do not differ and ask, what is the probability of a difference this large or larger if there is really no difference. If the answer is .05 or less, we call the result "statistically significant." But this is not really what we want to know.

It is useful to consider the question from a Bayesian perspective.[4] In the Bayesian approach, we ask, "What is the probability that the true effect is X, given our results?" rather than asking, "What is the probability of a result as large as ours if the true effect were zero?" The former question is more directly related to decisions we might make. When we apply the Bayesian approach, we ask about the probability of a wide range of effects, for example: "The reduction in HIV is 0"; "The reduction is 1 percent" "The reduction is 2 percent"—and so on. By calculating the probability of each effect size with Bayes's theorem, we can ask which has the highest probability. But, more important (usually), we can ask about the expected effect size. (For example, if effect sizes from 0 percent to 10 percent are all equally likely, and every other effect size has a probability of 0, then the expected effect size is 5 percent, the average.)

Bayes's theorem says that the probability of a given effect size ($p(H|D)$, the probability of the hypothesis H given the observed data D) is proportional to the probability of the data given that effect size ($p(D|H)$, the probability of the data given the hypothesis) times the prior probability of that effect size ($p(H)$). In other words, for the ith hypothesis H_i, $p(H_i)|D = cp(D|H_i)p(H_i)$, where c is a constant chosen to ensure that all probabilities add up to 1. The prior probability is the probability that we would assign to that effect before seeing the data.

Figure 8.1 shows a simplified example, in which we do not know the true proportion of an event (such as HIV cases) in a certain experimental condition. We start off with equal probabilities for each of eleven possible hypotheses (0, 0.1, 0.2, ..., 1.0). Then we observe 5 events out of 10 observations (the dashed line, e.g., 5 HIV cases out of 10 people in this experimental condition), or 50 out of 100 (solid line). The reason that the

---

[4]See Malakoff (1999) for a nontechnical introduction to Bayesian statistics.

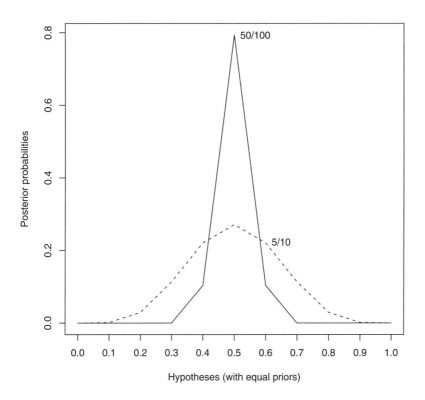

Figure 8.1: Effects of different sample sizes on posterior probabilities

lines are different is that the probability of exactly 50/100 is much higher given the hypothesis of 0.5 than given any other hypothesis. With only 10 observations, a result of 5/10 could happen with some substantial probability if the true proportion were 0.2 or 0.8.

Suppose that this were the effect of a drug, and we knew that, without the drug, the proportion of HIV cases was 0.7. The area to the left of 0.7 tells us how likely it is that the drug reduces the number of cases. Further, we might figure that, given the cost of the drug, anything over 0.6 is not worth it. So we really need to know how likely it is that the true effect of the drug is 0.6 or less, and this is quite a bit higher when we have more observations.

Figure 8.1 is based on the assumption that all of the eleven possible hypotheses examined were equally likely before data were collected. However, if we have reason to think that some are more likely than others—such as a prior study—we could take this information into account in our priors, and the posteriors would be higher for hypotheses that had higher priors. Of course, this procedure must be based on expert judgment, and judgment could be biased. But, if done properly, it could be a lot better than the assumption that all hypotheses are equally likely. The incorporation of human judgments into the priors is both controversial and promising, but it is not a necessary feature of the Bayesian approach.

At issue in the case of interest are three unknown parameters (numbers): K, the rate of transmission of HIV in the absence of treatment; L, the rate with the less expensive treatment; and M, the rate with the more expensive treatment. If the decision is between no treatment and the less expensive one, then we want to know $L - K$. If we have data from the two relevant groups—the less expensive treatment and the no-treatment control—then we can get a pretty good estimate of this difference, even if we do not use priors based on judgments.

On the other hand, if we are interested in $L - K$, and we do not have the no-treatment control, we must include some sort of prior distribution for K. If we assume that all possible values of K were equally likely, then information about L is not going to narrow the distribution of $L - K$ very much. Even if we knew that L is exactly 0.5, then $L - K$ would be equally likely to be anywhere between -0.5 (a harmful effect) and 0.5. Thus, we must include a judgment of K.

The use of the more expensive treatment as a control could help us make this judgment. We could, for example, have data from another country, where the more expensive treatment was compared to no treatment. We could assume that, in the country of interest, the effect of the more expensive treatment is proportionally about the same as in the data we have. For example, if a study in the United States showed that HIV transmission in some population of at-risk mothers declined from 20 percent to 5 percent with the more expensive treatment, and we observe a rate of 10 percent with the more expensive treatment in Uganda, we could assume that the no-treatment group would have roughly 40 percent transmission. But the key word here is *roughly*. There is no way to be sure, without actually running the no-treatment group. Moreover, there is no way to be sure about how much information we are losing by *not* testing this group, without relying on human judgment.

Now, in deciding whether to test a no-treatment condition, we may want to look at the costs and benefits of doing so. The costs, as noted, are largely the effect of this procedure on the recruitment of subjects for future studies. Surely, the use of active drugs in all arms of the study would make the researchers more popular, even if the no-treatment condition is not in itself a harm relative to no research at all. The benefits are a reduction in the number of subjects needed to get good results, hence the possibility of using the conclusions to help others more quickly. It is possible to estimate all these components of the analysis, but they all require judgment, including the effect of not using the no-treatment group.

Calculations of sample size that are based on traditional statistical methods typically ignore the question about what we really want to know. In particular, testing whether the less expensive and more expensive groups are "equal" does not allow us to determine the probability that either group is better than no treatment in the population of interest. Moreover, these two groups could be "not significantly different" yet still different enough so that the probability of exceeding some critical effect-size threshold is higher for the more expensive group than for the less expensive group (even taking into account the possibility that the thresholds are different because of the different costs).

In sum, the conclusion that an active control is statistically acceptable is based more on wishful thinking than on analysis in of the problem in terms of the decisions needed.

I should note, however, that there are other cases in which an active control is exactly right. More generally, the type of experiment to do should depend on the question at issue (Torrance, Drummond, and Walker 2003). I discuss this further in section 8.3.

8.2.2   Reducing the number of subjects

I should note that Bayesian methods are also capable of reducing the number of subjects needed in a clinical trial. At issue are the rules for stopping a trail. In the standard approach, as I discussed in section 8.2.1, the researcher gets the data and asks, "How likely is an effect as large as what I got if, in fact, there is no real effect?" This probability is called p. To calculate p, the research assumes a particular model for "no real effect." Usually, this model assumes that the measure of the effect has a normal (bell-shaped) distribution. The standard deviation of the distribution (a measure of subject-to-subject variability) can be estimated from the data. From the standard deviation and the difference between the means of the two groups, the researcher can calculate p. This model assumes that the number of subjects is fixed in advance.

Now suppose that the experimenter looks at the data every week and calculates p. Each week, some subjects will show positive effects and some will show negative effects. Because of this variation, p itself will vary up and down from week to week. Now suppose further that the researcher decides to stop the study when the result is "significant," which usually means when $p < .05$. The trouble is that the model used to calculate p does not take into account the weekly variation in p itself. The probability of getting a "significant" result in which $p < .05$ is really higher than .05, because the result could arise just from random variation in the p level. It is possible to correct for this, but then more subjects might be needed than in the stricter approach, in which the experimenter does not look at the data until the predetermined number of subjects are tested. Still, in general, looking often, applying the correction, and stopping when the corrected p level is significant can result in substantially fewer subjects than the fixed-sample approach. Despite this fact, the use of corrections is still rare, and more subjects are being tested than are really needed, even according to the traditional statistical model based on p levels.

The Bayesian approach can sometimes improve matters still further. Often, results that are nowhere near statistically "significant" can be useful for decision making, depending on what the decision is. For example, suppose you have a serious and rare disease, and your doctor says, "The only treatments for this disease are two medicines. The standard medicine has a 50 percent success rate. The new medicine is being tested, but, because the disease is rare, testing is slow, and you are going to have to decide before the results are available. The researchers who developed the new medicine were pretty sure that it is no worse than the standard one, but they were not at all sure that it is better. However, the new medicine has been successful in 4 of the 5 subjects who tried it." Now 4 out of 5 is not significantly different from 0.5. (In fact, $p = .18$.) But what would you do?

It hardly requires a formal Bayesian analysis to convince you that the new drug is very likely better than the old one. If you did need to estimate the probability, it would be reasonable to use the researchers' judgments as the basis of some priors. For example, you might assume that, for the eleven hypotheses considered in Figure 8.1, the prior probabilities are .01 for everything below 0.5, .05 for every point above it, and (hence) 0.7 for the hypothesis that the effect is 0.5. Then, the prior probability of being better than the standard drug is .25, and the posterior probability, after observing 4 out of 5 successes, is .38. The probability of being worse than the standard goes from .050 to .006. These changes might matter if there were some other reason not to try the new drug, such as side effects or cost.

8.2.3   Harm and benefit

The law requires research risks to be "reasonable" with respect to the anticipated benefits to the subjects (U. S. Government 1997). Placebo trials usually require greater risk to the subjects, but they usually require fewer subjects, at least to test the effectiveness of the treatment, as I have argued. As a result, a new drug will be available for patients quicker than in an active control design (Temple and Ellenberg 2000). In short, placebo-controlled trials present the problem of imposing harm on some patients for the benefit of other patients.

In general moral intuition opposes the idea of harming some to help others (Ritov and Baron 1990, Baron 1994, 1996b). For example, a hypothetical vaccine has a .05 percent chance of death from side effects but prevents a disease from which .10 percent will die. Although the net benefit of the vaccine warrants its use, many people oppose vaccination on the ground that the vaccine causes harm through the action of giving it. This effect has been called "omission bias." The term describes people's tendency to prefer harms caused by omission rather than those caused by action, relative to the decision that would yield the highest expected utility.

The standard response of the U.S. Food and Drug Administration and others is that the practice of placebo control is appropriate if the duration of the placebo is short and the potential harms (relative to an active control) are minimal (U.S. Food and Drug Administration 1989; Temple and Ellenberg 2000). Placebo controls are discouraged when the condition being treated is serious or life threatening. Thus, what matters is the balance of harm and benefit to the subjects of the research. An interesting feature of this practice concerning placebos is that they are acceptable when conditions are not very serious.

From the utilitarian perspective, this policy is difficult to justify, in general. It makes sense when the placebo condition requires subjects to forgo an effective treatment that they would otherwise get. Then, they really are at increased risk, and, unless they were adequately compensated for taking this risk, it would be irrational for them to take part in the study. They might be rationally willing to take small risks, however, for the benefit of others. When a study depends on irrational decisions for obtaining subjects, paternalism on the part of regulatory authorities seems justified.

But when the placebo condition is similar to the reservation option of not participating in the study, the control group is not at an "increased risk" relative to this alternative, so they might rationally do the study, even if they have assumed the worst case (having no chance of being in the experimental condition).

Moreover, aside from the problem of getting rational subjects to participate, a placebo study would seem (if anything) more warranted, in many cases, than an active-control study, because the placebo study can be done more quickly. In the situation for which the placebo condition is no better than not participating, there is apparently no good standard treatment. In this case, the more serious the disease, the more important it is to get the new drug to market quickly, if it turns out to work.

8.3   New drug approval

Currently in the United States, new drugs must be shown to be safe and effective. Approval comes in phases. First, the drug company submits an "investigational new drug" notice to the Food and Drug Administration (FDA). This must contain information about animal tests and other relevant data bearing on the issue of safety. It must also contain the plan for testing the drug on humans. Unless the FDA objects within 30 days, "phase I" studies on humans can begin. Phase I typically involves less than 100 subjects and takes about a year. The purpose is to find the appropriate dosage and to answer questions about how the body absorbs the drug. Phase II tests for side effects and effectiveness in a few hundred patients. It takes about another year. Phase III typically involves thousands of patients and can take two years or more. This is the main study of the drug's effectiveness and the most difficult part of the process, both financially and ethically. At the end of phase III, the company submits a "New Drug Application" to the FDA. The FDA is supposed to respond in 180 days, but it may ask for additional data. After approval of the drug, phase IV studies continue to monitor its effects and report data.

Consider the following situations:

1. The current situation   Drugs are illegal until they are tested against a placebo control. This makes it possible to attract subjects for drug trials with a placebo arm. The subjects (reasonably) think that the new drug might work and that they have a chance to get it. Those who do not get the drug are worse off than those who get it, if the drug is effective.

2. Initial legalization   Drugs are not prohibited. (False or misleading claims about them would be prohibited, but that is another issue.) When a promising new drug is first manufactured, patients would want it. In order to test its effectiveness, people would have to be paid to enter a trial in which they might *not* get the drug.

Intuitively (and I would suspect that most bioethicists would concur with this intuition) the second situation is bad because it would pay people to risk their health. The subjects in the placebo condition would not get the drug.

From a utilitarian perspective, the second situation is better for the subjects, however, if we assume that new drugs are, on the average, beneficial. More people get the drug in the second situation, specifically, everyone except those in the placebo condition. In the first situation, those who are not in the trial at all are also denied the drug. And in the second situation, subjects get paid more than they would in the first situation.

In fact, the United States has both situations coexisting. Dietary supplements and off-label uses of prescription drugs are both legal. Off-label use in particular has attracted attention because it serves as a kind of testing ground for what would happen if drugs were legal until they were banned rather than the other way around. Tabarrok (2000; see also Klein and Tabarrok 2004) has argued that the benefits of bringing drugs to market quickly outweigh the risks. Indeed, many off-label uses are for rare diseases and would never be brought to market at all if testing were required, because the tests would take so long. (See Madden [2004] for similar arguments.)

Another problem with new drug approval in the United States is that it requires no comparison of cost-effectiveness with current treatments. For approval, the drug must be safe and effective, even if it is much more expensive than an alternative that is just as good. Many new drugs are new treatments that are not clearly better than existing treatments for common disorders. Of course, it may be that these new "me too" drug are better for some patients, so perhaps they should be approved. (If new drugs were automatically approved, this would happen anyway.) Often, however, a new, more expensive drug is heavily advertised and is used even when it is no more effects. Comparative studies of both effectiveness and cost-effectiveness would reduce such wasteful expenditures (Goozner 2004).

8.4   Conclusion

I have suggested several ways in which drug development (one of the great achievements of the last century) could be even greater if it did not operate with one hand tied behind its back, sometimes with "ethics" holding the rope. We could pay subjects in order to move testing along more quickly. We could use subjects in poor countries, especially when the drugs being tested are designed to fight diseases of the world's poor. We could be less squeamish about placebo controls when they are warranted, and we could take advantage of modern statistical methods, both to reduce the required sample size overall and possibly also to avoid the use of placebo controls (and thus make subject recruitment easier). Finally, we could consider reducing the power of regulatory agencies to keep drugs off the market, while maintaining or increasing their power to certify information.

Major drug companies are often criticized for spending too much effort on the development of "me too" drugs that will generate income even if they do not get much market share. At the same time, the companies spend too little effort on drugs for diseases of poor people around the world, totally new kinds of drugs that could greatly benefit small groups of people in all countries (such as new cancer treatments), or new kinds of drugs that do not generate a steady income stream (such as new antibiotics), which are taken only for a short time by each patient.

One suggestion (in the *Economist*, Dec. 6, 2003, p. 14) is that governments regulate the price of new drugs according to an analysis of their benefit. Companies would be allowed to charge in proportion to the drug's benefit over the best available alternative. The argument is that most governments are already involved in the regulation of drug prices, but they use this regulatory power mostly to keep prices down, which conflicts with the goal of encouraging research. Under the proposed scheme, a beneficial new drug could be profitable as well, if the monetized benefit were greater than the cost of development and production.

Thus, the regulatory scheme would lead to some prices that were higher than those that the companies would charge in a free market—even with a patent. (Patents would still be needed.) "Me too" drugs would have very little additional benefit and would not be so lucrative.

This proposal would provide incentive for research on the most beneficial new drugs. It would, however, have the down side of raising drug prices for the poor. Thus, it would need to be coupled with some sort of help for the poor. That is, governments would have to pay the drug companies most of the designated price for drugs that poor people take.

Another less radical solution to the problem of "me too" drugs is for those who pay for most drugs—namely, insurers and governments—to encourage comparative testing, both for effectiveness and cost-effectiveness.

These solutions would work within a nation, but what about drugs for diseases such as tuberculosis and malaria, which now afflict mostly poor people in poor countries. Who will pay for them? And will they be included in the effectiveness analysis? I shall address these issues in the next chapter.

Chapter 9

Allocation

Questions about allocation of health care resources arise at all levels, from the world to the family. In general, the utilitarian approach to allocation holds that resources should be allocated so as to do the most good. Importantly, utilitarianism considers group boundaries as arbitrary (Singer 1982): nationalism is just as arbitrary as racism and sexism.[1] It also holds that future people count the same as present people, although we must also discount the future because of uncertainty, at least. The pure utilitarian view would lead to radical redistribution of resources, mostly from rich countries to poor ones, because most resources (such as money) provide more utility to the poor than to the rich.

In this chapter, for the most part, I shall emphasize another feature of the broad utilitarian approach, including decision analysis and economic analysis. It is capable of evaluating options as better or worse, and it can apply such evaluation to realistic options. Thus, rather than proposing a utopian vision and then trying to figure out how to get from here to there, I shall mostly deal with real options that policymakers face now. If we always choose the best options before us, then, eventually, we should come closer to utopia. Of course, it may be that this approach is too realistic. It may be better to refuse to help the poor, so that the revolution of the poor comes sooner. I shall not attempt such second guessing.

---

[1]This assumption is not unique to utilitarianism, of course, and it is also possible to apply utilitarianism to more limited domains.

9.1   Allocation heuristics and biases

In general, allocation "for the most good" is not the same as allocation based on intuitive judgment. Many of our judgments are based on principles of fairness that are very crude approximations to utility maximization. Such intuitive principles are sometimes built in to the law. These intuitions generally support policies that lead to worse consequences for some people—and potentially for everyone (Kaplow and Shavell 2002).

9.1.1   Omission bias

One kind of allocation bias (discussed in sections 3.1.2, 5.3, and chapter 8), is omission bias. This is the tendency to favor harms of omission over harms of action. It affects allocation because it inhibits the initiation of policies that increase harm to some while preventing more harm to others. An example is the near-removal from the market of a vaccine for pertussis (whooping cough) in the 1980s. The vaccine caused roughly the same disease it prevented, but the number of cases induced by the vaccine was far less than what would occur in an unvaccinated population. A similar, more recent example was the withdrawal of the rotavirus vaccine, which prevented a potentially deadly infection in infants (especially infants in poor countries) but also very rarely caused harmful side effects.[2] (Bazerman, Baron, and Shonk [2001] discuss these cases and others, such as the tendency of the U.S. Food and Drug Administration to worry more about approving harmful drugs than about failing to approve beneficial drugs.)

Ritov and Baron (1990) examined a set of hypothetical vaccination decisions modeled after such cases as these. In one experiment, subjects were told to imagine that their child had a 10 out of 10,000 chance of death from a flu epidemic. A vaccine could prevent the flu, but the vaccine itself could kill some number of children. Subjects were asked to indicate the maximum overall death rate for vaccinated children for which they would be willing to vaccinate their child. Most subjects answered well below 9 per 10,000. Of the subjects who showed this kind of reluctance, the mean tolerable risk was about 5 out of 10,000, half the

---

[2]See Roberts (2004) for some recent history.

risk of the illness itself. The results were also found when subjects were asked to take the position of a policymaker deciding for large numbers of children. When subjects were asked for justifications, some said that they would be responsible for any deaths caused by the vaccine, but they would be less responsible for deaths caused by failure to vaccinate.

In sum, "omission bias" is the tendency to judge the more harmful of two acts as worse when it is an act than when it is an omission, holding constant the differences in harm between the two acts (Baron and Ritov 1994). In any given case, some people display this bias and others do not.

Omission bias seems to be related to perceptions of physical causality. It is reduced when the action is an indirect cause of the harm, as opposed to a direct cause—for example, when an unvaccinated child gets a disease (Ritov and Baron 1990; Baron and Ritov 1994, Experiment 4; Royzman and Baron 2002; Spranca, Minsk, and Baron 1991), and it is highly correlated with judgments of causality. From a utilitarian perspective (and sometimes from a legal perspective) the relevant aspect of causality is control. If you could have behaved so as to prevent a bad outcome, then, in the relevant sense, you caused it (along with other causes). But the kind of causality that affects judgment when omission bias occurs is physical. There is a direct path between the action and the outcome.

Omission bias is somewhat labile. It can be reduced by the following kind of instructions (Baron 1992), which are illustrated for the vaccine case just described:[3]

> The questions you have just answered concern the distinction between actions and omissions. We would like you now to reconsider your answers....
>
> When we make a decision that affects mainly other people, we should try to look at it from their point of view. What matters to them, in these two cases, is whether they live or die.

---

[3]Of interest, this instruction influenced not only what people thought they should do but also whether they thought they would feel guiltier after vaccinating, if the bad outcome happened. People's expected emotions are correlated with their moral opinions, but the opinions seem to drive the expectations.

In the vaccination case, what matters is the probability of death. If you were the child, and if you could understand the situation, you would certainly prefer the lower probability of death. It would not matter to you how the probability came about.

In cases like these, you have the choice, and your choice affects what happens. It does not matter what would happen if you were not there. You are there. You must compare the effect of one option with the effect of the other. Whichever option you choose, you had a choice of taking the other option.

If the main effect of your choice is on others, shouldn't you choose the option that is least bad for them?

9.1.2   Protected values

People think that some of their values are protected from trade-offs with other values (Baron and Spranca 1997; Tetlock, Lerner, and Peterson 1996). Examples may include violations of the right to privacy or human reproductive cloning. People with protected values (PVs) against these things do not think they should be sacrificed for any compensating benefit, no matter how small the sacrifice or how large the benefit. In an economic sense, when values are protected, the marginal rate at which one good can substituted for another is infinite.

PVs concern rules about action, irrespective of their consequences. What counts as a type of action (e.g., lying) may be defined *partly* in terms of its consequence (false belief) or intended consequence. But the badness of the action is not just that of its consequences, so it has value of its own.

Omission bias is greater when PVs are involved (Ritov and Baron 1999). For example, when people have a PV for privacy, they are even less willing to violate privacy once in order to prevent several other violations. Thus, PVs apply to acts primarily, as opposed to omissions.

People think that their PVs should be honored even when their violation has no consequence at all. People who have PVs against the destruction of pristine forests, for example, say that they should not buy stock in a company that destroys forests, even if their purchase would not affect the share price and would not affect anyone else's behavior with respect to the forests. This is an "agent relative" obligation, a rule for the person holding the value that applies to his own choices but not (as much) to his obligations with respect to others' choices. So it is better for him not to buy the stock, even if his not buying it means that someone else will buy it.

PVs are at least somewhat insensitive to quantity. People tend to think it is just as bad to violate a PV once as it is to violate it several times (Ritov and Baron 1999).

Notice that the issue here is not behavior. Surely, people who endorse PVs violate them in their behavior, but these violations do not imply that the values are irrelevant for social policy. People may want public decisions to be based on the values they hold on reflection, whatever they do in their behavior. When people learn that they have violated some value they hold, they may regret their action rather than revising the value.

PVs may be seen as unreflective overgeneralizations. As such, they can be challenged. People can think of counterexamples to their own PVs. For example, they can think of values for which they might want to allow a pristine forest to be cut. When they think of such examples, they no longer say that they have a PV. Because PVs are mostly about actions rather than consequences, thinking of counterexamples also reduces omission bias (Baron and Leshner 2000).

9.1.3   Ex-ante equity

The terms *ex ante* and *ex post* refer respectively to before and after some uncertainty is resolved, for example, who will get a disease or a treatment. The ex ante bias is the finding that people want to equate ex ante risk within a population even when the ex post risk is worse (Ubel et al. 1996a). For example, many people would give a screening test to everyone in a group of patients covered by the same health maintenance organization (HMO) if the test would prevent 1,000 cancer cases rather than give a test to half of the patients (picked at random) that would prevent 1,200 cancer cases.

Ubel, Baron, and Asch (2001) found that this bias was reduced when the group was expanded. If subjects are told that the HMO actually covers two states and that the test cannot be given in one of the states, some subjects switched their preference to the test that prevented more cancers. It was as though they reasoned that, since the "group" was now larger, they could not give the test to "everyone" anyway. So they might as well aim for better consequences, given that "fairness" could not be achieved. This result illustrates a potential problem with some nonutilitarian concepts of distributive justice—namely, that the distributions they entail can change as the group definition is changed. If groups are arbitrary, then the idea of fair distribution is also arbitrary.

9.1.4   Proportionality and zero risk

People worry more about the proportion of risk reduced than about the number of people helped. This may be part of a more general confusion about quantities (section 3.2.1). The literature on the risk effects of pollutants and pharmaceuticals commonly reports relative risk, the ratio of the risk with the agent to the risk without it, rather than the difference. Yet, the difference between the two risks, not their ratio, is most relevant for decision making: if a baseline risk of injury is 1 in 1,000,000, then twice that risk is still insignificant; but if the risk is 1 in 3, a doubling matters much more.

Stone, Yates, and Parker (1994) found that relative risk information, as opposed to full information about the two absolute risks involved, made people more willing to pay for safety when risks were small. Fetherstonhaugh et al. (1997) found that people placed more value on saving lives when the lives saved were a larger proportion of those at risk. For example, subjects were told about two programs to save Rwandan refugees from cholera by providing clean water. The two programs cost about the same and both would save about 4,500 lives. One program would take place in a refugee camp with 250,000 refugees; the other, in a camp with 11,000. Subjects strongly preferred the program in the smaller camp.

I have suggested that these results were the result of quantitative confusion between relative risk and absolute risk (Baron 1997b). In one study, subjects expressed their willingness to pay (WTP) to reduce 18 causes of death (heart disease, stroke, chronic liver disease, and so forth) by 5 percent or by 2,600 people, in the United States. The typical (median) responses to these two questions correlated .96. Some causes of death were much more likely than others. For example, heart disease is about twenty times more likely than chronic liver disease as a cause of death. So 5 percent should not be a constant number for different causes. Still, subjects almost completely ignored the distinction between number of lives and percent of the problem. McDaniels (1988) found similar results for expenditures on risk reduction. His results paralleled actual expenditures, which tend to be greater (per life saved) for smaller risks.

If we can reduce risks to zero, then we do not have to worry about causing harm. This intuition is embodied in the infamous Delaney clause, part of a U.S. law, which outlawed any food additive that increases the risk of cancer by any amount (repealed after 30 years). Other laws favor complete risk reduction—such as the 1980 Superfund law in the United States, which concerns the cleanup of hazardous waste that has been left in the ground. Breyer (1993) has argued that most of the cleanup expenses go for "the last 10 percent" but that, for most purposes, the 90 percent cleanup is adequate. Cleanup costs are so high that it is proceeding very slowly. It is very likely that more waste could be cleaned up more quickly if the law and regulations did not encourage perfection.

The reduction of worry may, at first, seem to justify a zero-risk bias. Worry may increase greatly when the risk changes from zero to 1 percent, but it may not change much when the risk increases further. Thus, reduction to zero would have a disproportionate effect on worry. Although this argument may sometimes justify greater expenditures on reducing risks to zero, it does not do so when: (1) the risks are borne by others whose worry is unaffected by the decision; or (2) the risks reduced to zero are really parts of some larger risk, which remains, and which is the source of worry. Also, the disproportionate increase in worry when risks increase from zero, if it happens, may itself result from a proportionality bias. Better understanding of the quantitative nature of risk may result in a more linear increase in worry with increasing risk.

The zero-risk bias is found in questionnaires as well as in real life. In one questionnaire study, Baron, Gowda, and Kunreuther (1993) gave subjects the following case:

Two cities have landfills that affect the groundwater in the area. The larger city has 2,000,000 people, and the smaller city has 1,000,000. Leakage from the landfill in the larger city will cause 8 cases of cancer per year. Leakage from the landfill in the smaller city will cause 4 cases of cancer per year. Funds for cleanup are limited. The following options are available:

1. *Partially clean up both landfills.* The number of cancer cases would be reduced from 8 to 4 cases in the larger city and from 4 to 2 cases in the smaller city.

2. *Totally clean up the landfill in the smaller city and partially clean up the landfill in the larger city.* The number of cancer cases would be reduced from 8 to 7 cases in the larger city and from 4 to 0 cases in the smaller city.

3. *Concentrate on the landfill in the larger city, but partially clean up the landfill in the smaller city.* The number of cancer cases would be reduced to from 8 to 3 cases in the larger city and from 4 to 3 cases in the smaller city.

Although option 2 leads to a total reduction of 5 cases, and options 1 and 3 lead to a total of 6 cases, 42% of the subjects (who included judges and legislative aides) ranked option 2 as better than one of the others.

9.1.5   Marginal costs versus average cost

A similar bias concerns the way people think about costs. Economists evaluate changes at the margin—that is, in terms of the effects of increases and decreases. People may confuse marginal cost and average cost just as they confuse proportions and differences.

Kemp and Willetts (1995) found that subjects' ratings made little distinction among total utility of government services, utility per dollar spent, marginal utility per additional dollar, or utility per additional percent. All ratings were moderately correlated, to the same extent, with current expenditures, and highly correlated with each other.

Kemp and Willetts asked subjects to rate the value of government services in New Zealand, including items varying in the money spent on them, for example, government retirement income (NZ$4,314 million), universities (NZ\$577 million), and the New Zealand Symphony Orchestra (NZ\$8 million). Some subjects rated the usefulness per dollar spent, and others rated the total usefulness of each service, ignoring cost. Each subject rated both the overall utility (per dollar or total) and the marginal utility of an increase. In the per-dollar group, the marginal utility was "how useful or worthwhile you think each extra dollar spent on the item would be to New Zealand," and in the total group, the marginal utility was "how much value you think it would be to New Zealand if the government increased spending on the item by 5 percent." Subjects were not told the present cost of each service, but it would not be unreasonable for them to think that the amounts differed substantially.

We might expect that total utility would correlate with cost, while per-dollar utility would not correlate with cost. (Ideally, according to economic theory, per-dollar utility should be equal for all services.) In fact, both total and per-dollar ratings correlated moderately across services with log(cost) ($r = .55$ in both cases; correlations are based on mean ratings for each service across subjects). Subjects failed to distinguish between utility and utility per dollar.

Marginal-utility ratings should be uncorrelated with cost or with any other ratings, although we might expect positive correlations with cost for the marginal per-dollar ratings. Marginal ratings likewise correlated moderately with cost ($r = .41$ for total, .38 for per-dollar). Marginal ratings also correlated over $r = .90$ with total ratings in both conditions, and they correlated .99 with each other. In sum, subjects did not distinguish among different kinds of questions. Their ratings make more sense if we think of them as ratings of total utility, since the ratings were correlated with cost.

9.1.6   Matching versus maximizing

Several studies have presented subjects with allocation dilemmas of the following sort (Ubel and Loewenstein 1995, 1996a,b; Ubel et al. 1996b; Ubel, Baron, and Asch 1999): two groups of 100 people each are waiting for liver transplants. Members of group A have a 70 percent chance of survival after transplantation, and members of group B have a 30 percent chance. How should 100 livers—the total supply—be allocated between the two groups. The simple utilitarian answer is all to group A, but typically less than 20 percent of the subjects will choose this allocation. People want to give some livers to group B, even if less than half. Many want to give half. Some of this effect is the result of not knowing how to maximize. When subjects are asked what would maximize survival, some say that the allocation they chose would do so. But others make an explicit distinction between maximizing survival and being fair. They are willing to trade lives for fairness. Of course, the fairness is local. Others, perhaps those in other countries, are not in the scheme at all.

9.2   Allocation in practice

I have discussed some heuristics and biases in the abstract. I turn now to some specific issues that are affected by biases of the sort I have discussed.

9.2.1   Rationing

Health care is rationed everywhere. Even in the richest countries with the best insurance policies, health could be improved and lives saved by further expenditures that are not done. For example, we could have periodic whole body CAT scans to detect early cancer, or colonoscopies for everyone over 50, or over 45, which, if done often enough, could practically end deaths from colon cancer. We could spend more on health education, nutrition education, and mental health services. Most psychological depression still goes untreated, if only because people have not had sufficient education to recognize the symptoms, know that their condition is treatable, and seek help.

Of course, in poor countries, or for those lacking insurance in the few rich countries that do not provide it universally, the situation is more serious. People are living much shorter lives as a result of malaria, tuberculosis, and AIDS. The AIDS epidemic in Africa is on the edge of creating social breakdown in many areas because of the large number of orphans who are not being properly socialized.

Cost-effectiveness in Oregon

In the 1980s, the United States government provided funding for Medicaid, a government insurance program available to children and to those with incomes below the official poverty line. The benefits provided by Medicaid were comparable to those provided by private health insurance. But the program was not given enough funding to provide these benefits to all who qualified, let alone to the millions of others who were just above the poverty line but still found ordinary medical insurance too expensive.

To cope with this problem, the state of Oregon, led by John Kitzhaber (a doctor who became a state legislator and then governor), initiated the Oregon Health Plan, a program designed to provide Medicaid benefits to more people. In order to free up money for this extra coverage, the plan was to stop covering health services that were expensive and relatively ineffective, such as liver transplants that were unlikely to work anyway in people whose life expectancy was short—namely, older people. Thus, more people would get coverage for health care, but some people would do without very expensive procedures that did little good. Total utility would increase because the utility of the basic services provided to people would be very great, and the total loss to those who did without would be relatively small.

The state appointed a commission to elicit utility judgments from the public, with the idea of ranking condition-treatment pairs (treatment X for condition Y) in terms of cost-effectiveness. The state would then go down the list until it ran out of money, covering everything above this point. This way, the state would get the most total benefit for the dollars availalble. Notice that any switching above and below the line would make things worse. If some treatments below the line cost the same as some above it, then switching the two groups would mean that less benefit was obtained for the same cost.

Initially, opponents saw the plan as another way to pick on the poor, who were already picked on enough. Indeed, the very poor who qualified for Medicaid got a reduction in coverage. In 1987, Coby Howard, a seven-year-old boy, died of leukemia after being denied a bone-marrow transplant under Medicaid because the legislature had already decided not to cover such transplants. This was not part of the Oregon Health

Plan, but it raised fears of more of the same. This kind of treatment is exactly what would be cut off. It was very expensive and very unlikely to succeed. (Now the plan routinely covers such transplants.) But Kitzhaber and others rallied support for the plan, and it went ahead.

The commission made up a list of 709 condition-treatment pairs. Each pair was evaluated in terms of alleviation of symptoms, quality of life, and cost. To rate the utility of the symptoms, the commission conducted a telephone survey of Oregon residents. Each respondent rated 23 symptoms on a scale from 0 to 100, where 0 represents "as bad as death" and 100 represents "good health." The symptoms included such things as "burn over large areas of face, body, arms, or legs" (rated about half as bad as death), "trouble talking, such as lisp, stuttering, hoarseness, or inability to speak," and "breathing smog or unpleasant air" (rated closest to good health). The respondent also rated descriptions of limitations in mobility, physical activity, and social activity, such as health-related limitation in some social role.

Experts then used these ratings to determine the average benefit of each condition-treatment pair. They took into account the duration and probability of the benefits of treatment, compared to what would happen without the treatment under consideration. Then these benefits were divided by the cost to get the average benefit per dollar. Highest on the list were medical therapy for pneumonia and heart attacks. The lowest single item was life support for babies born without brains. The initial cutoff was set at 587. That is, the first 587 out of 709 items on the list would be covered. Items just above and below the cutoff, respectively, were treatment of cancer of the esophagus and breast reconstruction after mastectomy for cancer.

Public hearings led to major revisions in the list. People were disturbed to see that surgical treatment for ectopic pregnancy and for appendicitis were ranked about the same as dental caps for "pulp or near pulp exposure" in the list (Hadorn 1991). In fact, the expected benefit of tooth capping was 8 (on the scale of 0–100) and that of surgery for ectopic pregnancy was 71. The surgery is often lifesaving. People wanted a higher priority for potentially life saving treatments, and the list was revised in that direction. However, "If you want to check the results against your intuition, you should compare the *volumes* of different services that can be offered with a particular amount of resources. In this example, the appropriate comparison is not between treating a patient with dental caps for pulp exposure and treating a patient with surgery for ectopic pregnancy but between treating 105 patients with dental at $38 each versus treating one patient with surgery for ectopic pregnancy at $4,015 ($4,015/38 = 105$)" (Eddy 1991, p. 2138). On the other hand, the 8 versus 71 was the result of human judgment. If judgments are not as extreme as they should be, then the 8 was still too high, and the surgery should have ranked much higher.

In the end, the state implemented the plan, but the cutback in coverage was very small, only 2% of the total cost of the program (Jacobs, Marmor, and Oberlander 1999). Medicaid was extended to cover more poor people, but largely because of extra money from a cigarette tax and from other cost-saving measures. Many of the poor remain without coverage, although fewer than in other states. One fear that critics had was that the treatments below the line would still be highly beneficial for some patients, even though they were not beneficial on the average. These treatments are mostly provided, despite the rules.

The Oregon Health Plan is an example of what happens when the government sets out to ration health care in a way that maximizes utility. The problem is largely that the idea of rationing goes against people's intuitive judgments. Several sorts of judgments are at fault. Some involve the measurement of utilities. One possibility is that people exaggerate the seriousness of mild conditions. For example, Ubel et al. (1996) asked subjects, "You have a ganglion cyst on one hand. This cyst is a tiny bulge on top of one of the tendons in your hand. It does not disturb the function of your hand. You are able to do everything you could normally do, including activities that require strength or agility of the hand. However, occasionally you are aware of the bump on your hand, about the size of a pea. And once every month or so the cyst causes mild pain, which can be eliminated by taking an aspirin. On a scale from 0 to 100, where 0 is as bad as death and 100 is perfect health, how would you rate this condition?" The mean answer was 92. The cyst was judged about one-twelfth as bad as death. The ratio seems too large and the utility too far from 100. If the seriousness of minor conditions is overrated because of a distortion in the response scale, then these conditions will get higher priority in the final ranking than they deserve. People who look at the list would then want to move them down, and move more serious conditions up.

Baron and Ubel (2001) propose a second source of bias that could lead people to reject a cost-effectiveness ranking based on their utility judgments—the prominence effect (Tversky, Sattath, and Slovic 1988). When people make choices or examine rankings, they pay attention to the most prominent attribute of the available options, the attribute usually judged more "important," whereas, in judgment or matching tasks, they pay attention to all the relevant attributes. The utility judgments are all made under conditions that either do not involve trade-offs between health and cost at all or else encourage attention to both attributes of a treatment. When people look at a priority list, their desire to revise it could be based largely on the benefit, because benefit is the more prominent attribute. Just as cost is less prominent than benefit, it may also be true that the number of patients helped is less prominent than the amount of benefit per patient.

For a simple example, suppose treatment A costs $100 and yields an average of 0.01 QALY, therefore, costing $10,000 per QALY. And suppose treatment B costs $10,000 and yields 1 QALY, therefore having similar cost-effectiveness. Because of the different costs of each treatment, 100 people can receive treatment A for the same cost as providing one person with treatment B (in both cases yielding 1 QALY). A cost-effectiveness ranking would show these two treatments as being equally cost-effective. But, when evaluating such a ranking, people might focus primarily on the more prominent attribute—the amount of benefit brought by providing one person with each treatment—and, thus, they may want to move treatment B up higher on the list.

The practical implications are that either people should learn about this bias, or else they should not try to second-guess the results of cost-effectiveness analysis by tinkering with the rankings. Of course, tinkering is just what the Oregon commission could not resist doing. Perhaps, in the long run, the public will come to trust cost-effectiveness analysis even when it seems nonintuitive. Breyer (1993) and Sunstein (2002) have discussed how people might come to trust government regulatory bodies. Arguably, it is not impossible. Even now, people trust central banks to set monetary policy, and they trust professional organizations to make recommendations about medical treatments.

Bedside rationing

Who should decide to withhold some intervention on the ground that it is too expensive? I have assumed that the answer is "the insurer," whether this is a private company or the government. On this view, rich people would be allowed to pay for expensive treatments themselves. Or even not so rich people: The National Health in the U.K. does not cover bone marrow replacement for some cancers, and some "middle class" (i.e., comfortable but not wealthy) people pay for it themselves.

Ubel (2000) has argued that physicians are better able to make rationing decisions because they are able to take into account the patient's condition in more detail than simple rules would permit. If physicians persuaded their patients to forgo expensive or futile treatments, then the heavy hand of regulation (whether from the government or a company) would not be needed so much. Moreover, doctors would be in a better position to recognize when guidelines were inappropriate—for example, withholding an expensive treatment for arthritis in a patient who would benefit from it except that he is dying of cancer.

One problem with such bedside rationing, as Ubel recognizes, is that it affects the doctor-patient relationship. Many patients seem to expect their doctor to be an advocate for them against the forces of bureaucracy (although many do not; see Beach et al. 2003). In a system in which patients can choose doctors, doctors have an incentive to behave this way in order to keep their patients and avoid lawsuits. But, as Ubel (2000) argues, doctors face all kinds of incentives, including the incentive to overtreat when business is slow or to favor procedures for which reimbursement rates are better. Doctors must earn the trust of their patients within the limits that almost everyone faces, except perhaps judges with tenure.

Because bedside rationing is based on case-by-case judgments, it cannot be legislated or controlled. It must be part of a more general code of behavior that professionals try to follow. Because doctors have some incentive not to do it, we cannot expect too much of such a voluntary code. It can affect behavior only at the edges.

9.2.2 Organs

Some resources are scarce not just because they are expensive. The classic example is the supply of organs for transplantation. In most countries, the need for organs is far greater than the supply (see Bazerman, Baron, and Shonk 2001, ch. 1; Johnson and Goldstein 2003).

Of course, cost-effectiveness of transplantation varies from person to person. If we provide organs to the most needy recipients, then it might turn out that the cost-effectiveness for the rest is low. But this seems not to be the case. Kidney transplants, for example, seem to have great benefit, with cost-effectiveness improving over time and approaching $10,000 per life year (not quality adjusted in most studies; see Winkelmayer et al. 2002). Kidneys can also come from living donors, but those are also in short supply.

In fact, we do not quite go by cost-effectiveness. Organs are distributed by various formulas that take into account many factors—such as time on the waiting list. The formulas are not designed to maximize effectiveness. They take into account other factors such as giving priority to nearby recipients, seriousness of the recipient's condition, or time on the wait list.[4] These are factors that may be correlated with effectiveness, but that isn't the whole story about why they are considered. Seriousness of condition may sometimes work the other way: sicker patients may be less likely to survive a transplant. Time on the wait list may be a way of increasing the number of blacks who get transplants, who generally lose out statistically for a variety of reasons (Elster 1992, p. 115–117). And local priority may help encourage donation, on the assumption that people are more charitable toward those nearby. We also ignore factors that are relevant to predicting success, such as whether the recipient had a transplant already (Ubel, Arnold, and Caplan 1993). But the most important factors are those that predict success, such as close matches of antigens.

---

[4]See the Organ Procurement and Transplantation Network, at http://www.optn.org/, for examples of the rules.

Presumed consent for donation

Manipulations designed to increase donation might be unnecessary if more people were organ donors. If essentially everyone were willing to donate at their death, we then would be much closer to the point at which further increases in transplantation would not be cost-effective; perhaps we would even reach that point.

Data summarized by Johnson and Goldstein (2003) and Abade and Gay (2004) suggest that the "organ shortage" has essentially disappeared in some European countries, such as Belgium, where people are presumed to be organ donors unless they have explicitly opted out. This rule may change being a nondonor from a harmful omission to a harmful act, which seems worse (see section 9.1.1). It also puts inertia and indecision on the side of donating.

From a utilitarian perspective, this rule is clearly superior to the kind of opt-in rule used in most regions. The harm done to a potential recipient whose transplant is delayed can be very great. The harm done to donors is nonexistent in most cases. Most people really don't care that much about the integrity of their bodies after they die.

Some people care because of their particular religious beliefs. On the one hand, these beliefs can be harmful, hence worthy of discouraging or ignoring because of the effect they have on others. The more extreme cases are those in which parents are religiously opposed to medical care for their children, who suffer and die as a result. In a way, being a nondonor is similar in its effect. On the other hand, the history of religious persecution leads utilitarians to be cautious about acting on any judgment that goes against strong religious beliefs.

With presumed consent, we do take a risk that someone who really objects to donation will forget to opt out or be too embarrassed to do it (despite the excuse of strong religious beliefs, perhaps). So some harm results. The question is a comparison of magnitudes. In fact, two magnitudes: the magnitude of the harm to each person who either donates after death against her will or who suffers and dies prematurely while waiting for an organ; and the number of people in each category. The numbers are clearly on the side of presumed consent. It is difficult to judge the magnitudes, but, arguably, they are too.

Selling organs

> Should a poor man in Turkey or India be allowed to sell his
> kidney to a rich person in Israel or the United States, who
> needs a kidney and has the money to pay for it? This is a
> mutually advantageous exchange, but many serious writers
> have recommended against allowing such trade. To them this
> is an obnoxious market. To allow such a transaction is to of-
> fend human dignity....
>
> The indignity occurs in the fact of there being so much poverty
> that some people feel compelled to sell their body parts. That
> people actually sell their body parts is a mere manifestation
> of this systemic indignity. The indignity may cease to hit us
> in the face if such trades are not allowed. But they do not
> go away by virtue of this. In sum, if people are so poor that
> they need to trade their body parts, then we should encour-
> age policies to remove the poverty but not ban the trade.
>
> Basu (2002, 29–30)

Basu, in this passage, sums up the utilitarian view of this ugly situation. The same argument applies in other areas, such as the use of "cheap
labor" or the use of placebo control in poor countries (section 8.2). The
fact is that there is a market in organs of living people, and attempts to
discourage the practice simply drive up the price to the buyer and perhaps lower it to the seller (Finkel 2001).

It would be nice if the sellers had other ways to raise money. That
is the real problem, but it is a big problem that cannot be solved right
away. In the meantime, it would be nice if the sellers were better informed about the risks, and if operations were always performed in hospitals that provide the best care in cases of complications. (Sometimes
this happens, but rarely.) How could we at least get to this point?

It may help to increase the supply of organs. (I have addressed that
in the last section.) This would reduce the demand, lowering the price.
The price reduction would have two effects. One is that it would reduce
the attractiveness of raising money by selling an organ. The other, a
beneficial one, is that it would reduce the incentive that people have to
distort the risks when talking to a potential donor.

Public policies often have unintended side effects. But it does seem that a simple option that would help right away is to legalize and regulate organ donation for money. The regulation would insure that donors were not deceived in any way. Because much of the trade in organs is international, treaties may be required as well as laws.

9.2.3 Insurance

How should insurance rates and payoffs be set? In a way, this is an easy question for utilitarian theory, since it does not involve disgust reactions or a deep analysis of values. Yet, the theory of insurance is widely misunderstood. I shall argue for high deductables and copayments, and insurance premiums that largely ignore individual risk, except when they can provide incentives to promote better health. But insurance is part of a larger scheme of protection against risk, including the risk of poverty and its causes.

Insurance exists because of the declining marginal utility of money. Consider two types of people in a very simple situation. One person in a hundred needs a medical procedure that costs $100,000. Without insurance, that one person will suffer a large loss, which has a disutility, say, of 100. So that is the total utility loss for a hundred people. With insurance, the hundred people agree to pool their funds and pay for each other's operations. This means that each person loses $1,000, instead of one person losing $100,000. But the disutility of losing $1,000 is less than 1. It might be .5. This is because the loss of the $1,000 premium is "bearable." It means giving up the few last things that you would buy. But losing $100,000 means giving up "necessities," things that are really important. (It would mean borrowing, too, for most people.) Thus, the idea is to replace uncertain large losses with more predictable small losses. Insurance thus increases total utility by redistributing money from those who need it less to those who need it more by virtue of an unlucky event— that is, the need for an expensive procedure.

We also pay for the administrative costs of the insurance. When these costs are taken into account, insurance for small losses is not worth it. (This is why maintenance contracts on home appliances are rarely worthwhile for the consumer. The cost of a new washing machine is not that much greater than the cost of a contract for five years.) Yet, many insurance policies cover every doctor visit in full—every test, every procedure, and every prescription. The patient has no incentive to think twice before demanding such things, and waste surely occurs. That is called "moral hazard." People overuse services when insurance pays for them.

More generally, insurance pricing and rules can provide incentives. If we want to discourage smoking, we can increase the cost of health insurance for smokers.

If health insurance is universal, what should it pay for? The clear answer is that it should pay for the most catastrophic needs, but not the nickel-and-dime stuff. It should be unlimited at the high end but have deductable and copayment amounts at the low end. The administrative costs alone make it inefficient for insurance to reimburse people for every doctor visit and every prescription.

Moral hazard provides another reason against small payments. People should have to pay what they can "easily lose" toward any medical service that they get. The precise rules need to be calculated, but it is clear that very few insurance policies—health or other kinds—follow this principle. Many have limits on the *maximum* they will pay; such limits defeat the purpose of insurance. And many reimburse every dollar for some things, wastefully because of the administrative costs alone (including the time involved in submitting claims). The fact that it is impossible even to buy automobile insurance in many U. S. states with more than $500 deductable suggests that both consumers and insurers are missing the boat (especially because the same policies often have limits at the high end).

If deductables and copayments were included in all insurance, the poor would suffer, because the money would have more utility to them, even small amounts of money. But other kinds of subsidies could help the poor more efficiently, subsidies that did not encourage waste.

If health insurance is universal, what should it cost? The simple answer is that it should cost the same for each person for each year. But this has an immediate problem: Old people require more medical care. If everyone paid the same, then those who die young would apparently subsidize those who live long enough to take full advantage of health insurance in their old age. Is this a problem? The question is, if annual costs were equal regardless of age, can we increase total utility by taking from the old and giving to the young? The reasons that come to mind in favor of such a policy are not specific to health: the old are usually richer. If that is true, then the solution is to tax the rich and help the poor. Adjusting health insurance rates for age would be crude way to obtain the benefits of redistributive taxation. On the other hand, if redistribution through taxation is insufficient, then some good can be done by increasing the cost of insurance for old people. But, on the other hand again, old people are less able to work, so taking money from them does not have the incentive effect that it has on younger people. In general, the utilitarian arguments for higher costs for the old are not very strong. Similar arguments apply for differential rates for men and women. It seems that no benefit results from charging one gender more than the other, even if one gender uses more services than the other.

Another reason to charge different rates is to provide incentives. This provides a reason to charge more to smokers, heavy drinkers, and the obese—but only if the prospect of higher rates can provide sufficient incentive to change. All of these behaviors are only partly under the control of incentives. In economic terms, the elasticity of demand for cigarettes, excessive food, or alcohol is low.

Universal insurance is better than optional insurance from a utilitarian perspective. People in developed countries who are not covered by insurance usually do not pay fully for their health care. They throw themselves at the mercy of others and usually get it. As a result, they get care that costs more than it should—for example, because it is provided in emergency rooms—and that is less effective, to the point of increasing death rates (Doyle 2005).

Since everyone has universal insurance, the question of how it should be paid for is simply part of the larger question about the distribution of income. In other words, what matters is the ultimate distribution. We could have everyone pay a flat fee and then make up for it through a negative income tax. Or we could have people pay on a sliding scale and achieve the same result. Politically, it may matter, because people may favor or oppose something that is called a tax rather than a premium. But that is all.

It is conceivable that optional insurance could maximize utility. For example, automobile insurance is optional, because people do not have to drive. Automobile insurance thus provides some incentive not to drive. It makes people pay the full cost of their decision to drive. But this is not the case for health insurance. There is nothing anyone can do to avoid the possibility of illness.

What if insurance is not universal? Then a different concern comes into play. Insurance premiums must be designed to make each person willing to buy the insurance. This means that rates must be tailored to risk. Young people must pay less than old people, and healthy people must pay less than those with heart disease, diabetes, and other chronic conditions, or risk factors such as genetic predispositions to cancer. These are things that people can know. If you know that you are low risk, with none of these factors, insurance may not be a good deal for you. This phenomena is called "adverse selection." Those at higher risk will buy insurance, and those at lower risk will not. Insurance companies, knowing that this happens, will charge higher rates than they would charge if insurance were universal. If they did not charge higher rates, they would lose money.

Various laws and proposed laws are designed to prevent insurance companies from denying insurance to those at higher risk, for example, for reasons knowable through genetic tests (Rothenberg and Terry 2002). The effect of these laws is to make it possible for individuals to know more about their risks than insurance companies know (or can use). These laws will lead to adverse selection and higher rates, unless insurance is universal, because the people who know they are least at risk will not buy insurance, and the insurance companies will have to raise rates to cover the costs of their remaining high-risk clients. It is not clear that the laws do more good than harm. A complex calculation would be required to tell. The real problem is the continued possibility of opting out of health insurance.

Why insure just health? Well, we don't. Advanced countries also insure people against acquired disability, and people can purchase private disability insurance and insurance against early death—life insurance. When such insurance is privately purchased and optional, we have the problem of adverse selection again (Nowlan 2002).

But why stop with such a limited set of offerings? Many sources of luck affect our lives. Shiller (2003) has argued that the idea of insurance can be extended in a variety of ways through new financial instruments that spread risk. In the limit, why couldn't we all have insurance before we are born against the kinds of problems that would lead us to poverty or relative poverty? Since we cannot purchase it, the market has failed, and government must intervene by taxing us in order to provide it. A world government could provide insurance against being born in a poor country, perhaps the biggest risk of all, and totally beyond one's control.

This is, of course, a utopian fantasy of the sort I said I would avoid, but it is perhaps a useful way to think about redistribution—namely, as a kind of compulsory insurance that government provides because the market cannot provide it.

9.3   What to do about biases

In this chapter and elsewhere in this book (and in Baron 1998, and Bazerman, Baron, and Shonk 2001), I have discussed several biases in decision making that affect public policy when they play out in the political domain. These biases are held by citizens, politicians, government officials, and other policy makers (such as hospital administrators and insurance executives). Their effect cannot be reduced by simply changing the power balance among these groups. Here I briefly review the alternatives for reducing such biases, or the harm that results from them.

First, it is sometimes possible to teach people to respond with reduced biases. This is found both in short-term laboratory studies and in studies of the effects of training in relevant disciplines such as statistics or economics (Larrick 2004). Even a single course in statistics can reduce biases in problems related to the course.

Kahneman and Frederick (2002) provide an interesting analysis of de-biasing in terms of two systems, which they call intuitive and reflective. Many biases arise in the intuitive system. People have learned (or evolved) to make fast judgments on the basis of cues (attributes) that are statistically useful but often misleading. The reflective system can learn to override these quick, intuitive judgments. Some biases are demonstrated as inconsistencies between judgments of two cases. For example, in one classic case discussed in the article, subjects given a description of Linda as having been a politically active college student were asked whether Linda is now more likely to be "a bank teller" or "a bank teller active in the feminist movement." The second category is included in the first, so it cannot be more probable. Yet, subjects judged the second category as more probable. This happened with college-student subjects as well as experts in statistics, so long as the two categories were separated from each other so that their relationship was not obvious. When the two categories were put right next to each other, however, the college students still made the error, but the experts did not. This finding illustrates the possibility of training the reflective system to override the response of the intuitive system, provided that the reflective system can discover the problem. It also shows that training can sometimes help.

Results such as these argue for increased education at all levels in the basic principles of decision theory. These principles overlap almost completely with the basic principles of probability, statistics, and microeconomics. These are useful topics in their own right, which may deserve more attention in the high school curriculum and on the tests that students take when they apply to university. (More attention on the tests would affect secondary schools in short order.) Some of the principles can even be taught before secondary school (Baron and Brown 1991). Increased education will lead to greater understanding of the role of experts and expert knowledge (Baron 1993b).

Notice, though, that most of the biases discussed here are elicited in transparent cases. They are indications of the failures of the reflective system. In some cases, people feel committed to their answers. (The same is true for subjects who respond to the transparent version of problems such as Linda.) If these commitments have already developed before some educational intervention is attempted, it may be too late. Some people with commitments like these may become philosophers, and they may use all the tools of their trade to defend their original commitments.

Ultimately, though, individual citizens are not going to determine the details of health policy. Perhaps politicians should not attempt it either. Following the suggestions of Breyer (1993) and Sunstein (2002), we might imagine that allocation of health resources be studied by a central agency. The role of this agency could vary from nation to nation, and there could also be an international agency to examine world allocation. In the United States, we might imagine that the agency would apply decision analysis to make recommendations. It could work collaboratively with outside groups—for example, those associated with professional organizations such as the American College of Obstetricians and Gynecologists[5]—just as the U.S. Food and Drug Administration works with outside researchers to evaluate drugs. The judgments of such an agency might be binding on some programs (such as those run by government itself) but advisory for other programs (such as insurance companies).

What is crucial in a democracy is that a critical mass of citizens be able to understand what such an agency is doing. By analogy, the determination of interest rates was once a matter for politicians, and it was often debated in political campaigns. Now, most countries "know better." The United States, for example, has turned the matter over to an agency comprised of economic experts, the Federal Reserve. Enough citizens seem to have sufficient understanding of what this agency is doing so that it retains the trust of voters and politicians alike, who tend to leave it alone. Some education has been necessary for this, but not a lot. Citizens are still fairly ignorant about macroeconomic theory.

9.4   Conclusion

Often, our intuitive judgments are allocations based on heuristic principles that yield good results but may also fail to yield the best results overall. We tend to focus on what is salient—such as acts as opposed to omissions, or *ex ante* equity as opposed to *ex post*, proportions as opposed to differences, and average cost as opposed to marginal cost. We elevate principles to the status of absolutes, failing to think of exceptions. Such judgments express themselves as policies, not because of any insidious takeover of the policy process but by general agreement. The allocation of organs and health insurance are examples.

Education can increase people's understanding of the economic principles of allocation. Citizens do not need to know how to make the calculations themselves in order to appreciate the idea of maximizing the benefits per dollar. Likewise, education may encourage legislators to resist the temptation to fine-tune the allocation of health resources themselves. Instead, they may find it useful to rely on specialized agencies, which they supervise in a general way.

The biggest problems of allocation are, however, on the world level. That is the topic of the next chapter.

---

[5]http://acog.org.

Chapter 10

The Bigger Picture

From a utilitarian perspective—and, indeed, from many others—national and group boundaries are not themselves relevant to questions about how we allocate goods. Of course, boundaries can affect our options at a given time. A national legislature usually cannot make laws that apply to residents of other countries, and an insurance company cannot by itself set policies for other companies. Still, when we start thinking about opportunities to do good or avoid harm—that is, to increase utility—the low-hanging fruit has to do with world distribution, possibly distribution over time, and distribution between rich and poor within nations. We can do more good, more cheaply by fighting AIDS and malaria in Africa than by fussing over consent forms for research studies.

10.1   The politics of improving world health

Ophthalmologists in Norway provide excellent care, but there are too few of them. Waiting lists are long, and some patients are never seen at all (Elster 1993). The overall result would be better if care were a bit less thorough so that more patients could be seen. Elster refers to a "norm of thoroughness" to describe the heuristic that justifies the present system. The idea is to give those who get into the system the same high level of care. Something analogous happens when nations provide extensive (and expensive) health care for residents but not for nonresidents.

My complaint here is not against the idea of equality. When utility is marginally declining, and when we do not depend on inequality for incentive, we can essentially always increase total utility by reducing inequality, even within a local area. The problem is rather the near-total neglect of non-nationals in the formation of public policy.

It is easier and less costly to improve health in Africa than it is to do so in Europe or the United States (although the lack of universal insurance in the United States means that some easy things can be done here too; see Pauly 2002; Physicians' Working Group for Single-Payer National Health Insurance 2003). Poor countries have higher rates of serious diseases that can be prevented with relative ease (compared to the big killers in rich countries)—such as malaria, tuberculosis, AIDS, and malnutrition—which exacerbates other problems. Many scholars have argued that it is efficient to spend money to improve health beyond the money that is spent trying to improve economic conditions in general, since health is an input to economic development (see, e.g., Sachs 2001).

The neglect of these problems is everywhere. Foreign aid is minimal, despite some posturing and promising. Research done by drug companies is largely directed at new drugs for chronic diseases of those who can pay, which do not include most of the world's poor. Agricultural research, which might help alleviate malnutrition, is also minimally concerned with the problems of food production in the poorest countries. Research funding from governments of rich countries is also largely designed to help with problems faced by the citizens of those countries.

One might argue that this is understandable, because nations are concerned about themselves. But nations are not people. Advanced democracies are designed to carry out the voters' will, more or less. If a candidate for United States president runs for office promising a massive "Marshall Plan" to lift the poor nations of the world out of poverty,[1] a utilitarian who believed the candidate's commitment might well vote for such a candidate, on the ground that she would do the most good. A utilitarian voter has no obligation to put the utility of conationals above the utilities of others. His only concern is to do the most good through his political action.

---

[1] In Bazerman, Baron, and Shonk (2001, ch. 6), we outlined a program that could be put into effect with minimal sacrifice.

Real voters are *parochial*. They tend to put conationals ahead of others. Parochialism is a strong and basic psychological phenomenon. It can be observed even in small, arbitrary, groups of people who do not know each other (Baron 2001).

One might argue that voters vote out of self-interest, hence vote for the good of their nation. But, if they rationally pursue their self-interest, they would not vote at all. It isn't worthwhile. Most voters do seem to vote out of a sense of trying to do the most good, as they see it (see Edlin, Gelman, and Kaplan 2003). That is why so few voters throw away their votes by voting for candidates that have no chance.

Part of the problem is that voters—and political actors in general—may be confused about what they are doing. They may partly believe that they are defending their self-interest and that voting works like a market in which everyone has equal purchasing power, and hence equal influence over the supply of goods. This story is consistent with the idea that minorities need constitutional protection, lest the goods they want are not produced at all. I have suggested other confusions, however (Baron 1997c, 2001).

First, parochialism may result from illusions in which people think that cooperation with their own group is in their self-interest. They may think, "I am just like everyone else in my group. If I vote for what is best, then so will others" (Quattrone and Tversky 1984). It is true that people are subject to common influences, but that does not mean that they influence each other very much.

A second type of illusion is the "illusion of morality as self-interest" (Baron 1997c). People seem to deny the existence of the conflict between self and others, the conflict that defines a social dilemma. Because morality and self-interest are usually correlated, people tend to overgeneralize and act as though the two are correlated even when they are not. Thus, people think that contributing to a public good is in their self-interest, even though it is not.

The self-interest illusion can encourage cooperation, and this is a good thing when cooperation should be encouraged. However, it can also encourage cooperation that benefits one's group at the expense of outsiders. People who sacrifice on behalf of others similar to themselves may be more prone to the self-interest illusion, because they see the benefits as going to people who are like themselves in some salient way. They think, roughly, "My cooperation helps people who are X. I am X. There-fore, it helps me." This kind of reasoning is easier to engage in when X represents a particular group than when it represents people in general.[2]

Baron (2001) found that this illusion is indeed greater when groups are competing. Moreover, when the subjects had to calculate their gains and losses, the tendency to favor their own group decreased. The results on the whole suggest that one determinant of parochialism is that the self-interest illusion is greater when an in-group is in competition with an out-group. The contrast between two competing groups increases the perceived similarity between the decision maker and the other group members, thus increasing the tendency to think that "anything that helps the group helps me, because I am like them."

This effect is somewhat labile. As suggested by Singer (1982), it may be possible, through reason, to understand the arbitrariness of group boundaries. The more people think of boundaries as arbitrary, the more they can direct their non-self-interested concern at the greater good rath-er than the parochial interests of their group.

10.2 Environment, animals, and future people

The "bio" in bioethics includes the biosphere in general. Our actions affect animals and plants, and they affect the environment that we pass on to future living things, including people. How do we think about the utility effects of decisions that affect the biosphere over the long term?

Singer (1993, ch. 10) explains the basic utilitarian view, as I under-stand it. Nature has no utility as such, except insofar as it affects the utilities of sentient beings. People have values for protecting the natural environment. Insofar as these values are real—that is, insofar as they are not means values based on false beliefs—they count.

Singer also counts the pleasures and pains of animals. This is a diffi-cult issue that I shall leave aside after pointing out some problems. Caus-

---

[2]Of course, this sort of reasoning contains a germ of truth. If we hold constant the gross cost of cooperation to the individual and the total benefit of cooperation to the group, then the net cost of cooperation (gross cost minus the cooperator's share of the group benefit) is smaller when the group is smaller. Also, in real life, people can influence each other more when the group is smaller. The illusion goes beyond this germ of truth, however.

ing pain in animals is bad. Killing them is not so bad as killing people because, to a first approximation, they have no plans of the sort that people have. One utilitarian view is that animals are replaceable: all that matters is the total utility of their experiences, so killing one and replacing it with another has no net effect. But this position implies that more animals are always better, provided that their lives are better than not existing. We might escape this problem by applying the same reasoning that I have applied to human population: the issue comes down to our goals for the creation of goals. But, if we do this, we are apparently free to do anything to animals but cause them pain, since pain depends on the goals of existing animals. Singer, a committed defender of animal rights and vegetarianism, would certainly disagree with this conclusion. As I said, I do not want to get into this issue here.

Similar paradoxes arise in thinking about the future (see Portney and Weyant 1999). We have several reasons to discount the future. The main one, perhaps, is that we are uncertain about the effects of our choices on future events, and this is more true, when the events are farther away in time. The history of efforts to forecast the future of economic development or technology beyond a few years, does not inspire much confidence. If our uncertainty can be described as concerning random events that occur with equal probability over time (such as new inventions or environmental catastrophes), then we should discount according to an exponential function (i.e., the value of the future declines by a constant fraction of its starting value in each time period). This is also the function we use when we calculate the value of future money, assuming a constant rate of interest.

Another reason to discount the utilities of future people is that it might be harder for us to increase them, at least by giving them more money. The average material standard of living has been steadily increasing. Thus, future people will be better off, and the usual utilitarian rationale for redistribution implies that utility would increase if we take from them and give to ourselves. In the absence of any reason to assume otherwise, exponential discounting is a reasonable assumption here.

When we think about monetary expenditures, still another reason to discount the future is interest itself. If we invest money instead of spending it, it will increase over time, and we can do more good by spending it in the future. That is usually the alternative option to spending money now for things that benefit the future. If we spend now on behalf of the future, we must make sure that we can do more good for future people than we could do by simply investing the money and passing it on to them. This reason also suggests exponential discounting.

Now we run into a problem. If we discount the future exponentially, it still doesn't go away. If we think about the value of endangered species to people—and a substantial fraction of all species seem to be endangered—the value may not be very high, but it goes on and on. The integral of a declining exponential function is the logarithmic function, which has no asymptote. It goes up and up forever. This means that the preservation of endangered species could have a much greater value than we are giving it, to put it mildly. That is because a species, once lost, is presumably lost forever.

Although I have no solution to this problem, I can perhaps say something more relevant to the present context. Future people count. This matters when we consider the benefits of medical research in particular. Unlike the benefits of species preservation, these benefits will not go on forever, since new technologies tend to be superseded at some point. But we may tend to forget future people when we think about the costs and benefits of research.

10.3   Waste

In discussions about allocation of health goods, we often find ourselves thinking, "Wouldn't it be nice to have more money for X?" where X could be many different things. Rarely do we think that it would be nice to spend less money on something. Yet, money—and, more generally, resources—are finite. The money must come from somewhere. Politicians usually say they will "reduce waste." They usually mean waste in whatever governmental unit they want to control. In health policy, we think about money wasted on unnecessary surgery, frivolous doctor visits, and drugs that have no more benefits than (much cheaper) placebos.

In a utilitarian perspective, however, the waste that is reduced need not come from something related to the place where the money is needed. We could, for example, tax luxuries and spend the money on vaccinations. Although people generally do prefer matching of sources to expenditures (see, e.g., Beattie and Baron 1995), the tax system can be used to reduce waste in many different areas, by taxing it.

For all the railing of anti-tax activists against government waste, they rarely point to it. When government waste is obvious, as in the case of farm subsidies, the savings from reducing it are usually small in the big scheme of things. Arguably, the low-hanging fruit, when it comes to waste, is in the area of private expenditures. When we look at the utility per dollar of many positional goods and luxury goods, it seems low (Frank 1999).

A simple solution to reduce such waste has been proposed by Edward McCaffery (2001, 2002), who argues for a progressive consumption tax in place of the income tax used in many countries (as discussed in section 4.1.4). McCaffery does not emphasize utilitarian arguments, but they are easy to make. The idea is that the utility per dollar spent each year by each person declines as a function of the amount spent. This follows from a kind of minimal criterion of rationality: people spend money first on the things they need the most—that is, the things with the highest utility per dollar. Thus, it makes sense to allow each person some amount of expenditure (such as $20,000, tax free) on the assumption that this money will be spent on goods that ought to be available to everyone. (Income of poor people could be supplemented in order to bring them up to this level, or they could be given in-kind goods and services.) Then a moderate tax would kick in until some higher level of expenditure was reached, and then a very high tax would take effect. People with high incomes who lived frugally would not be taxed much, but the money would be taxed later, whenever it was spent.

This system has several advantages over some of the obvious alternatives. One is that government does not need to decide what is a luxury and what is wasteful. McCaffery's proposal leaves that question to the rational decisions of individuals. Another advantage is that, unlike the otherwise similar sales tax or value-added tax, this tax is progressive and retains the redistributive function of a progressive income tax. Although it could be said that the idea encourages savings, it could also be said that the progressiveness would allow the nearly poor to spend more on basic goods.

Another simple solution, not incompatible with McCaffery's, is to tax negative externalities, such as pollution. When we take into account the social costs of pollution, it is clearly wasteful, because it yields less utility per dollar than other comparable uses of resources.

My point, so far, is that we can reduce waste in many ways other than by cutting expenditures on health care. But we can reduce waste easily in health care too. A simple way to do that is to use deductables and copayments in health insurance, whether the insurance is provided by government or by private companies, as I argued in section 9.2.3.

10.4   Conclusion

I have argued that many of the real decisions that appeal to bioethics for their justification are influenced by intuitive heuristics and biases, which arise without much reflection about ultimate purposes and justifications. These include naturalism, bias toward harms of omission as opposed to those of action, confusion of coercion with predictability of choice, elevation of rules of thumb to absolutes (such as the necessity of consent or equality in allocation), and confusions about quantitative issues in allocation (such as proportions versus differences and matching versus maximizing).

In the present chapter, I also continued an argument made elsewhere in this book that the intuitive appeal to bioethical principles leads to a kind of disproportionate, penny-wise and pound-foolish emphasis on minor problems involving flat maxima, while ignoring major problems such as the problems of the poor.

I have argued that a different approach to these problems will yield better outcomes overall. The different approach involves the application of decision analysis based on consequences, which I call utilitarian decision analysis, because it adds up changes in utility over people. In some cases, this kind of analysis can be used explicitly by experts who have the necessary time and knowledge. In other cases, its basic principles, such as the maximization of benefits per dollar spent, can be understood by enough people with sufficient education so that policies approximating the implications of the analysis can be put in place and receive sufficient political support as to be stable.

I thus advocate greater reliance on experts in decision analysis, such as those who belong to the Decision Analysis Society or the Society for

Medical Decision Making,[3] as well as experts in economic analysis.

Utilitarian decision analysis teaches us some general lessons about decision making, even if the mathematical aspects are put aside:

- Think quantitatively. We can do this even without assigning numbers. We can think about where to put our effort so as to maximize its benefits without putting numbers on the benefits.

- Compare options. Choice depends on the difference between the two best options. The status quo, the default option, and the ideal world are (by themselves) irrelevant.

- Consider the future. It is future consequences that matter, not sunk costs. Of course, past events (such as promises) affect future consequences, but it is those consequences that matter.

- Consider psychological effects. In contrast to naive economic theory (of a sort that most economists don't use anymore), utilitarian decision theory considers subjective outcomes.

- Combine utilities. The big idea of utilitarianism is that we can combine utilities across outcomes of different kinds that affect different people. Our natural tendency is to isolate effects, thinking of one at a time, sometimes focusing one effect, sometimes on another.

Three things will happen if bioethics moves in the direction I have tried to illustrate. First, it will become more technical. It will provide more analyses of decisions in terms of probabilities and utilities. More generally, it will consider trade-offs. If we require such and such, what do we give up? What are the costs?

Second, it will change its focus. It will be less concerned with issues of rights and more concerned with issues that affect the health and well-being of large numbers of people in major ways (Varmus et al. 2003). Issues of world health will come to the fore.

Third, we might expect government and institutional regulations to be more libertarian and less moralistic (section 3.1.4). Bioethics will not be so much a matter of telling us what desires we ought to have. In particular, it will not be about telling us that our desire to live long, or to reproduce—whatever it takes to do so—are false.

---

[3]See http://faculty.fuqua.duke.edu/daweb/ and http://www.smdm.org.

References

Abade, A. and Gay, S. (2004). The impact of presumed consent legislation on cadaveric organ donation: A cross country study. Kennedy School of Government Research Working Paper RWP04–024 `http://ssrn.com/abstract=562841`.

Alger, A. (1999). Trials and tribulations. *Forbes Magazine*, May 17.

Angell, M. (1997). The ethics of clinical research in the Third World. *New England Journal of Medicine, 337*, 847–849.

Appelbaum, P. S., Grisso, T., Frank, E., O'Donnell, S., and Kupfer, D. J. (1999). Competence of depressed patients for consent to research. *American Journal of Psychiatry, 156*, 1380–1384.

Aquinas, Thomas (1947). *Summa Theologica.* (Translated by the Fathers of the English Dominican Province.) Benziger Brothers. Inc. `http://www.newadvent.org/summa/`

Baron, J. (1992). The effect of normative beliefs on anticipated emotions. *Journal of Personality and Social Psychology, 63*, 320–330.

Baron, J. (1993a). *Morality and rational choice.* Dordrecht: Kluwer.

Baron, J. (1993b). Why teach thinking?—An essay. (Target article with commentary.) *Applied Psychology: An International Review, 42*, 191–237.

Baron, J. (1994). Nonconsequentialist decisions (with commentary and reply). *Behavioral and Brain Sciences, 17*, 1–42.

Baron, J. (1996a). Norm-endorsement utilitarianism and the nature of utility. *Economics and Philosophy, 12*, 165–182.

Baron, J. (1996b). Do no harm. In D. M. Messick and A. E. Tenbrunsel (Eds.), *Codes of conduct: Behavioral research into business ethics*, pp. 197–213. New York: Russell Sage Foundation.

Baron, J. (1997a). Political action vs. voluntarism in social dilemmas and aid for the needy. *Rationality and Society, 9*, 307–326.

Baron, J. (1997b). Confusion of relative and absolute risk in valuation. *Journal of Risk and Uncertainty, 14*, 301–309.

Baron, J. (1997c). The illusion of morality as self-interest: a reason to cooperate in social dilemmas. *Psychological Science, 8*, 330–335.

Baron, J. (1998). *Judgment misguided: Intuition and error in public decision making.* Oxford: Oxford University Press.

Baron, J. (2000). *Thinking and deciding* (3d ed.). New York: Cambridge University Press.

Baron, J. (2001). Confusion of group-interest and self-interest in parochial cooperation on behalf of a group. *Journal of Conflict Resolution, 45*, 283–296.

Baron, J. (2003). Value analysis of political behavior—self-interested : moralistic :: altruistic : moral. *University of Pennsylvania Law Review, 151*, 1135–1167.

Baron, J., Asch, D. A., Fagerlin, A., Jepson, C., Loewenstein, G., Riis, J., Stineman, M. G., and Ubel, P. A. (2003). Effect of assessment method on the discrepancy between judgments of health disorders people have and do not have: A Web study. *Medical Decision Making, 23*, 422–434.

Baron, J., and Brown, R. V. (Eds.) (1991). *Teaching decision making to adolescents.* Hillsdale, NJ: Erlbaum.

Baron, J., Gowda, R., and Kunreuther, H. C. (1993). Attitudes toward managing hazardous waste: What should be cleaned up and who should pay for it? *Risk Analysis, 13*, 183–192.

Baron, J., Hershey, J.C., and Kunreuther, H. (2000). Determinants of priority for risk reduction: The role of worry. *Risk Analysis, 20*, 413–427.

Baron, J., Lawson, G., and Siegel, L. S. (1975). Effects of training and set size on children's judgments of number and length. *Developmental Psychology, 11*, 583–588.

Baron, J., and Leshner, S. (2000). How serious are expressions of protected values. *Journal of Experimental Psychology: Applied, 6*, 183–194.

Baron, J., and Ritov, I. (1993). Intuitions about penalties and compensation in the context of tort law. *Journal of Risk and Uncertainty, 7*, 17–33.

Baron, J., and Ritov, I. (1994). Reference points and omission bias. *Organizational Behavior and Human Decision Processes, 59*, 475–498.

Baron, J., and Ritov, I. (2005). Head vs. heart: The role of emotions in judgments about policies. Draft, University of Pennsylvania.

Baron, J., and Spranca, M. (1997). Protected values. *Organizational Behavior and Human Decision Processes, 70*, 1–16.

Baron, J., and Ubel, P. A. (2001). Revising a priority list based on cost-effectiveness: The role of the prominence effect and distorted utility judgments. *Medical Decision Making, 21*, 278–287.

Basu, K. (2002). Sexual harassment in the workplace: An economic analysis with implications for worker rights and labor standards policy. MIT Department of Economics Working Paper, 02–11. `http://people.cornell.edu/pages/kb40/`

Bazerman, M. H., Baron, J., and Shonk, K. (2001). *You can't enlarge the pie: The psychology of ineffective government.* New York: Basic Books.

Bazerman, M.H., Morgan, K.P. and Loewenstein, G. (1997). The impossibility of auditor independence. *Sloan Management Review, 38*, 89-94.

Beach, M. C., Asch, D. A., Jepson, C., Hershey, J. C., Mohr, T., McMorrow, S., and Ubel, P. A. (2003). Public response to cost-quality tradeoffs in clinical decisions. *Medical Decision Making, 23*, 369–378.

Beattie, J. and Baron, J. (1995). In-kind vs. out-of-kind penalties: Preference and valuation. *Journal of Experimental Psychology: Applied, 1*, 136–151.

Beattie, J., Baron, J., Hershey, J. C., and Spranca, M. (1994). Determinants of decision seeking and decision aversion. *Journal of Behavioral Decision Making, 7*, 129–144.

Beauchamp, T. L., and Childress, J. F. (1983). *Principles of biomedical ethics* (2nd ed.). New York: Oxford University Press.

Behn, R. D., and Vaupel, J. W. (1982). *Quick analysis for busy decision makers.* New York: Basic Books.

Bohnet, I., Frey, B. S., and Huck, S. (2001). More order with less law: On contract enforcement, trust, and crowding. *American Political Science Review, 95*, 131–144.

Bown, N., Read, D., and Summers, B. (2003). The lure of choice. *Journal of Behavioral Decision Making, 16*, 297–308.

Brennan, T. A., Sox, C. M., and Burstin, H. R. (1996). Relation between negligent adverse events and the outcomes of medical-malpractice litigation. *New England Journal of Medicine, 335*, 1963–1967.

Breyer, S. (1993). *Breaking the vicious circle: Toward effective risk regulation.* Cambridge, MA: Harvard University Press.

Broome, J. (1991). *Weighing goods: Equality, uncertainty and time.* Oxford: Basil Blackwell.

Cain, D. M., Loewenstein, G., and Moore, D. A. (2005). The dirt on coming clean: Perverse effects of disclosing conflicts of interest. *Journal of Legal Studies.*

Calabresi, G. (1970). *The costs of accidents: A legal and economic analysis.* New Haven: Yale University Press.

Callahan, D. (2003). *What price better health? Hazards of the research imperative.* Berkeley, CA: University of California Press.

Camerer, C. F., Issacharoff, S., Loewenstein, G., O'Donoghue, T., and Rabin, M. (2003). Regulation for conservatives: Behavioral economics and the case for "asymmetric paternalism." *University of Pennsylvania Law Review, 151,* 1211–1254.

Caplan, A. L. (1992). *If I were a rich man could I buy a pancreas?: and other essays on medical ethics.* Bloomington, IN: Indiana University Press.

Casarett, D., Karlawish, J., and Asch, D. A. (2002). Paying hypertension research subjects. *Journal of General Internal Medicine, 17,* 650–652.

Chivers, M. L., Rieger, G., Latty, E., and Bailey, J. M. (2004). A sex difference in the specificity of sexual arousal. *Psychological Science, 15,* 736–744..

Chomsky, N. (1957). *Syntactic structures.* The Hague: Mouton.

Cohen, J. (1997). Ethics of AZT studies in poorer countries attacked. *Science, 276,* 1022.

Connor, E. M., Sperling, R. S., Gelber, R., Kiselev, P., Scott, G., O'Sullivan, M. J., VanDyke, R., Bey, M., Shearer, W., Jacobson, R. L., Jimenez, E., O'Neill, E., Bazin, B., Delfraissy, J.-F., Culnane, M., Coombs, R., Elkins, M., Moye, J., Stratton, P., Balsley, J., The Pediatric AIDS Clinical Trials Group Protocol 076 Study Group (1994). Reduction of maternal-infant transmission of human immunodeficiency virus type 1 with zidovudine treatment. *New England Journal of Medicine, 331,* 1173–1180.

Coppolino, M. and Ackerson, L. (2001). Do surrogate decision makers provide accurate consent for intensive care research? *Chest, 119,* 603–612.

Cronbach, L. and Snow, R. (1977). *Aptitudes and Instructional Methods: A Handbook for Research on Interactions*. New York: Irvington.

Dawes, R. M., Faust, D., and Meehl, P. E. (1989). Clinical versus actuarial judgment. *Science, 243*, 1668–1674.

Dawes, R. M., Orbell, J. M., Simmons, R. T., and van de Kragt, A. J. C. (1986). Organizing groups for collective action. *American Political Science Review, 80*, 1171–1185.

Deber, R. B., and Goel, V. (1990). Using explicit decision rules to manage issues of justice, risk, and ethics in decision analysis. *Medical Decision Making, 10*, 181–194.

de Finetti, B. (1937). Foresight: Its logical laws, its subjective sources. (Translated by H. E. Kyburg, Jr., and H. E. Smokler.) In H. E. Kyburg, Jr., and H. E. Smokler (Eds.) *Studies in subjective probability.* New York: Wiley, 1964.

DeKay, M. L., and Asch, D. A. (1998). Is the defensive use of diagnostic tests good for patients, or bad? *Medical Decision Making, 18*, 19–28.

Djankov, S. D., La Porta, R., De Silanes, F. L., and Shleifer, A. (2000). The regulation of entry. Harvard Institute of Economic Research Paper No. 1904.

Doyle, J. J. (2005). Health insurance, treatment, and outcomes: Using auto accidents as health shocks. NBER Working Paper No. 11099. `http://www.nber.org/papers/w11099`

Easterbrook, G. (1995). *A moment on the earth: The coming age of environmental optimism*. New York: Viking.

Eddy, D. M. (1991). Oregon's methods: Did cost-effectiveness analysis fail? *Journal of the American Medical Association, 266*, 2135–2141.

Edlin, A., Gelman, A., and Kaplan, N. (2003). Rational voting and voter turnout. Unpublished article, Columbia University. `http://www.stat.columbia.edu/~gelman/phd.students/rational4.ps`

Eichenwald, K. and Kolata, G. (1999). Drug trials hid conflicts for doctors. *New York Times*, May 16, A1, A34–35.

Elster, J. (1983). *Sour grapes: Studies of the subversion of rationality*. New York: Cambridge University Press.

Elster, J. (1992). *Local justice: How institutions allocate scarce goods and necessary burdens*. New York: Russell Sage Foundation.

Elster, J. (1993). Justice and the allocation of scarce resources. In B. A. Mellers and J. Baron (Eds.), *Psychological perspectives on justice: The-*

ory and applications (pp. 259–278). New York: Cambridge University Press.

Entorf, H., Feger, J., and Kölch, M. (2004). Children in need of medical intervention. ZEW Discussion Paper No. 04–49. `ftp://ftp.zew.de/pub/zew-docs/dp/dp0449.pdf`.

Etchells, E., Darzins, P., Silberfeld, M., Singer, P. A., McKenny, J., Naglie, G., Katz, M., Guyatt, G. H., Molloy, D. W., and Strang, D. (1999) Assessment of patient capacity to consent to treatment. *Journal of General Internal Medicine, 14,* 27–34.

Fairchild, A. L. and Bayer, R. (1999). Uses and abuses of Tuskegee. *Science, 284,* 919–921.

Falk, A. (2004). Distrust—the hidden cost of control. IZA Discussion Paper No. 1203. `http://www.iza.org/home/falk`

Farah, M. (2002). Emerging ethical issues in neuroscience. *Nature Neuroscience, 5,* 1123–1129.

Fazel, S., Hope, T., and Jacoby, R. (1999). Assessment of competence to complete advance directives: validation of a patient centred approach. *British Medical Journal, 318,* 493–497.

Fehr, E. and Gächter, S. (2000). Fairness and retaliation: the economics of reciprocity. *Journal of Economic Perspectives, 14,* 159–181.

Fehr, E. and Rockenbach, B. (2003). Detrimental effects of sanctions on human altruism. *Nature, 422,* 137–140.

Fetherstonhaugh, D., Slovic, P., Johnson, S., and Friedrich, J. (1997). Insensitivity to the value of human life: A study of psychophysical numbing. *Journal of Risk and Uncertainty, 14,* 283–300.

Finkel, M. (2001). Complications. *New York Times Magazine* (section 6), May 27, pp. 26 ff.

Finnis, J. (1980). *Natural law and natural rights.* Oxford: Clarendon.

Foster, K. R. and Vecchia, P. (Eds.) (2002–3). Special issue on the precautionary principle. *IEEE Technology and Society Magazine, 21* (4).

Frank. R. H. (1999). *Luxury fever: Why money fails to satisfy in an era of excess.* New York: Free Press.

Frey, B. and Jegen, R. (2001). Motivation crowding theory. *Journal of Economic Surveys, 15,* 589–611.

Frey, B. S. and Oberholzer-Gee, F. (1997). The cost of price incentives: An empirical analysis of motivation crowding-out. *American Economic Review, 87,* 746–755.

Ganiats, T. G. (1996). Justifying prenatal screening and genetic amnio-centesis programs by cost-effectiveness analysis. *Medical Decision Making, 16*, 45–50.

Goozner, M. (2004). *The $800 million pill: The truth behind the cost of new drugs*. Berkeley, CA: University of California Press.

Grady, C. (2001). Money for research participation: Does it jeopardize informed consent? [with commentary] *American Journal of Bioethics, 1*, 40–67.

Greene, J. and Baron, J. (2001). Intuitions about declining marginal utility. *Journal of Behavioral Decision Making, 14*, 243–255.

Hadorn, D. C. (1991). Setting health care priorities in Oregon: Cost-effectiveness meets the rule of rescue. *Journal of the American Medical Association, 265*, 2218–2225.

Haidt, J. and Hersh, M. (2001). Sexual morality: The cultures and reasons of liberals and conservatives. *Journal of Applied Social Psychology, 31*, 191–221.

Hamburger, P. (2005). The new censorship: Institutional review boards. (May 2005). University of Chicago, Public Law Working Paper No. 95. http://ssrn.com/abstract=721363

Hare, R. M. (1952). *The language of morals*. Oxford: Oxford University Press.

Hare, R. M. (1963). *Freedom and reason*. Oxford: Oxford University Press.

Hare, R. M. (1981). *Moral thinking: Its levels, method and point*. Oxford: Oxford University Press.

Harsanyi, J. C. (1953). Cardinal utility in welfare economics and in the theory of risk taking. *Journal of Political Economy, 61*, 454–435.

Henrion, M. and Fischhoff, B. (1986). Assessing uncertainty in physical constants. *American Journal of Physics, 54*, 791–798.

Hertwig, R. and Ortmann, A. (2001). Experimental practices in economics: A methodological challenge for psychologists? *Behavioral and Brain Sciences, 24*, 383–403.

Hirsch, F. (1976). *Social limits to growth*. Cambridge, MA: Harvard University Press.

Hoeyer, K. and Lynöe, N. (2004). Is informed consent a solution to contractual problems? A comment on the article ' "Iceland Inc."?: On the Ethics of Commercial Population Genomics' by Jon F. Merz, Glenn E. McGee, and Pamela Sankar. *Social Science and Medicine, 58*, 1211.

Holden, C. and Vogel, G. (2004). A technical fix for an ethical bind? [News Focus]. *Science, 306*, 2174–2176.

Hunink, M., Glasziou, P., Siegel, J., Weeks, J., Pliskin, J., Elstein, A. S., and Weinstein, M. C. (2001). *Decision making in health and medicine: Integrating evidence and values.* New York: Cambridge University Press.

Iyengar, S. S. and Lepper, M. (2000). When choice is demotivating: Can one desire too much of a good thing? *Journal of Personality and Social Psychology, 79*, 995–1006.

Iyengar, S. S. and Lepper, M. R. (2002). Choice and its consequences: On the costs and benefits of self-determination. In A. Tesser, and D. A. Stapel (Eds.), *Self and motivation: Emerging psychological perspectives.* (pp. 71-96). Washington, DC: American Psychological Association.

Jacobs L., Marmor T., and Oberlander J. (1999). The Oregon Health Plan and the political paradox of rationing: What advocates and critics have claimed and what Oregon did. *Journal of Health Politics, Policy and Law, 24*, 161–80.

Jenni, K. E. and Loewenstein, G. (1997). Explaining the"identifiable victim effect." *Journal of Risk and Uncertainty, 14*, 235–257.

Jervis, R. (1976). *Perception and misperception in international politics.* Princeton: Princeton University Press.

Johnson, E. J. and Goldstein, D. (2003). Do Defaults Save Lives? *Science, 302*, 1338–1339.

Jones-Lee, M. W. (1992). Paternalistic altruism and the value of statistical life. *Economic Journal, 102*, 80–90.

Juengst, E. T., Binstock, R. H., Mehlman, M. J., and Post, S. G. (2003). Antiaging research and the need for public dialogue. *Science 299*, 1323.

Kahneman, D. and Frederick, S. (2002). Representativeness revisited: Attribute substitution in intuitive judgment. In T. Gilovich, D. Griffin, and D. Kahneman (Eds.), *Heuristics and biases: The psychology of intuitive judgment*, pp. 49–81.

Kahneman, D., Frederickson, B. L., Schreiber, C. A., and Redelmeier, D. A. (1993). When more pain is preferred to less: Adding a better end. *Psychological Science, 4*, 401-405.

Kahneman, D. and Tversky, A. (2000). *Choices, values, and frames.* New York: Cambridge University Press (and Russell Sage Foundation).

Kant, I. (1983). *Grounding for the metaphysics of morals.* In I. Kant, *Ethical philosophy*, trans. James W. Ellington. Indianapolis: Hackett (originally published 1785).

Kaplow, L. and Shavell, S. (2002). *Fairness versus welfare.* Cambridge, MA: Harvard University Press.

Karlawish, J. H. (in press). Emergency research. In E. Emanuel, D. Grady, and D. Wendler (Eds.). *Oxford textbook of research ethics.* New York: Oxford University Press.

Karlawish, J. H. T., Casarett, D. J., and James, B. D. (2002). Alzheimer's disease patients' and caregivers' capacity, competency, and reasons to enroll in an early-phase Alzheimer's disease clinical trial. *Journal of the American Geriatrics Society, 50,* 2019–2024.

Keeney, R. L. (1992). *Value-focused thinking: A path to creative decisionmaking.* Cambridge, MA: Harvard University Press.

Keeney, R. L. and Raiffa, H. (1993). *Decisions with multiple objectives: Preference and value tradeoffs.* New York: Cambridge University Press. (Originally published, 1976.)

Kemp, S. and Willetts, K. (1995). Rating the value of government-funded services: comparison of methods. *Journal of Economic Psychology, 16,* 1–21.

Kessler, D. P. and McClellan, M. B. (2002). How liability law affects medical productivity. *Journal of Health Economics, 21,* 931–955.

Kim, S. Y. H., Caine, E. D., Currier, G. W., Leibovici, A., and Ryan, J. M. (2001). Assessing the competence of persons with Alzheimer's disease in providing informed consent for participation in research. *American Journal of Psychiatry, 158,* 712–717.

Kim, S. Y. H., Karlawish, J. H. T., and Caine, E. D. (2002). Current state of research on decision- making competence of cognitively impaired elderly persons. *American Journal of Geriatric Psychiatry, 10,* 151–165.

Klein, D. B. and Tabarrok, A. T. (2004). Who certifies off-label? *Regulation,* Summer, pp. 60–63.

Köbberling, V. and Wakker, P. P. (2003). A simple tool for qualitatively testing, quantitatively measuring, and normatively justifying Savage's expected utility. *Journal of Risk and Uncertainty, 28,* 135–145.

Krantz, D. H., Luce, R. D., Suppes, P., and Tversky, A. (1971). *Foundations of measurement* (Vol. 1). New York: Academic Press.

Kuppermann, M. Goldberg J. D., and Nease R. F Jr. Washington A. E. (1999). Who should be offered prenatal diagnosis? The 35-year-old question. *American Journal of Public Health, 89,* 160–163.

Kuppermann, M., Nease R. F., Jr., Learman, L. A., Gates, E., Blumberg, B., and Washington A. E. (2000). Procedure-related miscarriages and Down syndrome-affected births: Implications for prenatal testing based on women's preferences. *Obstetrics and Gynecology, 96* 511–516.

Larrick, R. P. (2004). Debiasing. In D. J. Koehler and N. Harvey (Eds.), *Blackwell Handbook of Judgment and Decision Making*, pp. 316–337. London: Blackwell.

Lawson, G., Baron, J., and Siegel, L. S. (1974). The role of length and number cues in children's quantitative judgments. *Child Development, 45*, 731–736.

Ledley, R. S. and Lusted, L. B. (1959). Reasoning foundations of medical diagnosis. *Science, 130*, 9–21.

Lemmens, T. and Miller, P. B. (2003). The human subjects trade: Ethical and legal issues surrounding recruitment incentives. *Journal of Law, Medicine, and Ethics, 31*, 398–418.

Lepper, M. R. and Greene, D. (Eds.). (1978). *The hidden costs of reward.* Hillsdale, NJ: Erlbaum.

Lichtenberg, F. R. (2002). Sources of U.S. longevity increase, 1960–1997. NBER Working Paper No. W8755. Cambridge, MA: National Bureau of Economic Research. http://www.nber.org

Lichtenberg, F. R. (2004). The expanding pharmaceutical arsenal in the war on cancer. NBER Working Paper No. W10328. Cambridge, MA: National Bureau of Economic Research http://www.nber.org.

Localio, A. R., Lawthers, A. G., Brennan, T. A., Laird, N. M., Hebert, L. E., Peterson, L. M., Newhouse, J. P., Weiler, P. C., and Hiatt, H. H. (1991). Relation between malpractice claims and adverse events due to negligence: Results of the Harvard Medical Practice Study III. *New England Journal of Medicine, 325*, 245–251.

Lurie, P. and Wolfe, S. (1997). Unethical trials of interventions to reduce perinatal transmission of the human immunodeficiency virus in developing countries. *New England Journal of Medicine, 337*, 853–856.

Madden, B. J. (2004). Breaking the FDA monopoly. *Regulation*, Summer, pp. 64–66.

Malakoff, D. (1999). Bayes offers a "new" way to make sense of numbers. *Science, 286*, 1460–1464.

McCaffery, E. J. (2001). Must we have the right to waste? In S. Munzer (Ed.), *New Essays in the Legal and Political Theory of Property.* New York:

Cambridge University Press.

McCaffery, E. J. (2002). *Fair not flat: How to make the tax system better and simpler.* Chicago: University of Chicago Press.

McDaniels, T. L. (1988). Comparing expressed and revealed preferences for risk reduction: Different hazards and question frames. *Risk Analysis, 8,* 593–604.

Merz, J. F., McGee, G. E., and Sankar, P. (2004). "Iceland, Inc."?: On the ethics of commercial population genomics. *Social Science and Medicine, 58,* 1201–1209.

Miller, H. I. (2000). Gene therapy on trial. (Letter.) *Science, 287,* 591.

Miller, R. A. (2002). Extending life: Scientific prospects and political obstacles. *Millbank Quarterly, 80,* 155–174.

Mueller, J. H. and Fuerdy, J. J. (2001). Reviewing the risk: What's the evidence that it works? *APS Observer (American Psychological Society), 14* (7), 1, 26–38, and (8) 19–20.

National Commission for the Protection of Human Subjects of Biomedical and Behavioral Research (1979). *The Belmont Report: Ethical Principles and Guidelines for the Protection of Human Subjects of Research.* Washington, DC: U. S. Food and Drug Administration. `http://www.fda.gov/oc/oha/IRB/toc11.html`

Nease, R. F. Jr. Kneeland, T., O'Connor, G. T., Sumner, W., Lumpkins, C., Shaw, L., Pryor, D., and Sox, H. C. (1995). Variation in patient utilities for outcomes of the management of chronic stable angina. Implications for clinical practice guidelines. *Journal of the American Medical Association, 273,* 1185–90.

Nease, R. F., Jr. and Owens, D. K. (1994). A method for estimating the cost-effectiveness of incorporating patient preferences into practice guidelines. *Medical Decision Making, 14,* 382–392.

Nichol, G., Huszti, E., Rokosh, J., Dumbrell, A., McGowan, J., and Becker, L. (2003). Impact of informed consent requirements on cardiac arrest research in the United States: Exception from consent or from research? *Academic Emergency Medicine, 10,* 534.

Nowlan, W. (2002). A rational view of insurance and genetic discrimination. *Science, 297,* 195–196.

Oliver, A. (2004). Prioritizing health care: Is "health" always an appropriate maximand? *Medical Decision Making, 24,* 272–280.

Pascal, B. (1941). *The provincial letters.* New York: Random House (originally published 1656).

Pauly, M. V. (2002). Why the United States does not have universal health insurance: a public finance and public choice perspective. *Public Finance Review, 30,* 349–365.

Physicians' Working Group for Single-Payer National Health Insurance. (2003). Proposal of the Physicians' Working group for Single-Payer National Health Insurance. *Journal of the American Medical Association, 290,* 798–805.

Plous, S. and Herzog, H. (2001). Reliability of protocol reviews for animal research. *Science, 293,* 608–609.

Popper, K. R. (1962). Why are the calculi of logic and arithmetic applicable to reality? Chapter 9 in *Conjectures and refutations: The growth of scientific knowledge,* pp. 201–214. New York: Basic Books.

Portney, P. R. and Weyant, J. P. (Eds.) (1999). *Discounting and intergenerational equity.* Washington: Resources for the Future.

President's Council on Bioethics. (2002). *Human cloning and human dignity: An ethical inquiry.* Washington, DC. `http://bioethics.gov/reports/cloningreport/`

President's Council on Bioethics. (2003). *Beyond therapy: Biotechnology and the pursuit of happiness.* Washington, DC. `http://bioethics.gov/reports/beyondtherapy/`

Quattrone, G. A. and Tversky, A. (1984). Causal versus diagnostic contingencies: On self-deception and the voter's illusion. *Journal of Personality and Social Psychology, 46,* 237–248.

Quinn, W. (1989). Actions, intentions, and consequences: The doctrine of double effect. *Philosophy and Public Affairs, 18,* 334351.

Raiffa, H. (1968). *Decision analysis.* Reading, MA: Addison-Wesley.

Ramsey, F. P. (1931). Truth and probability. In R. B. Braithwaite (Ed.), *The foundations of mathematics and other logical essays by F. P. Ramsey* (pp. 158–198). New York: Harcourt, Brace.

Rapoport, J. L., Buchsbaum, M. S., Weingartner, H., Zahn, T. P., Ludlow, C., and Mikkelsen, E. J. (1980). Dextroamphetamine. Its cognitive and behavioral effects in normal and hyperactive boys and normal men. *Archives of General Psychiatry, 37,* 933–943

Rapoport, J. L., Buchsbaum, M. S., Zahn, T. P., Weingartner, H., Ludlow, C., and Mikkelsen, E. J. (1978). Dextroamphetamine: cognitive and behavioral effects in normal prepubertal boys. *Science, 199*, 560–563.

Rawls, J. (1971). *A theory of justice.* Cambridge, MA: Harvard University Press.

Ritov, I. and Baron, J. (1990). Reluctance to vaccinate: omission bias and ambiguity. *Journal of Behavioral Decision Making, 3*, 263–277.

Ritov, I. and Baron, J. (1999). Protected values and omission bias. *Organizational Behavior and Human Decision Processes, 79*, 79–94.

Roberts, L. (2004). Rotavirus vaccine's second chance [News Focus]. *Science, 305*, 1890–1893.

Rothenberg, K. H. and Terry, S. F. (2002). Before it's too late—addressing fear of genetic information. *Science, 297*, 196–197.

Rothman, D. J. (2000). The shame of medical research. *New York Review of Books, 47*, 60–64.

Royzman, E. B. and Baron, J. (2002). The preference for indirect harm. *Social Justice Research.*

Rubin, P. H. (2005). The FDA's antibiotic resistance. *Regulation, 27*, Winter, 34–37.

Sachs, J. D. (2001). Tropical underdevelopment. NBER Working Paper No. w8119. Cambridge, MA: National Bureau of Economic Research. http://www.nber.org.

Savage, L. J. (1954). *The foundations of statistics.* New York: Wiley.

Schwartz, B., Ward, A., Monterosso, J., Lyubomirsky, S., White, K., and Lehman, D. R. (2002). Maximizing versus satisficing: Happiness is a matter of choice. *Journal of Personality and Social Psychology, 83*, 1178–1197.

Schweitzer, M. E. and Ho, T. (2004). Trust but verify: Monitoring in interdependent relationships. http://ssrn.com/abstract=524802

Shavell, S. M. (1987). *Economic analysis of accident law.* Cambridge, MA: Harvard University Press.

Shavell, S. M. (2004) *Foundations of economic analysis of law.* Cambridge, MA: Harvard University Press.

Shiller, R. J. (2003). *The new financial order: Risk in the 21st century.* Princeton, NJ: Princeton University Press.

Sidgwick, H. (1962). *The methods of ethics. (7th ed., 1907)* Chicago: University of Chicago Press. (First edition published 1874).

Sieber, J. E., Plattner, S., and Rubin, P. (2002). How (not) to regulate social and behavioral research. *Professional Ethics Report (American Associa-*

tion for the Advancement of Science), 15, 1–4. http://www.aaas.org/spp/sfrl/per/per29.htm

Singer, P. (1982). *The expanding circle: Ethics and sociobiology.* New York: Farrar, Strauss and Giroux.

Singer, P. (1993). *Practical ethics* (2nd ed.). Cambridge: Cambridge University Press.

Smithline, H. A. and Gerstle, M. L. (1998). Waiver of informed consent: a survey of emergency medicine patients. *American Journal of Emergency Medicine, 16,* 90–1.

Spranca, M., Minsk, E., and Baron, J. (1991). Omission and commission in judgment and choice. *Journal of Experimental Social Psychology, 27,* 76–105.

Stolberg, S. G. (1999). The biotech death of Jesse Gelsinger. *New York Times Magazine,* November 28.

Stone, E. R., Yates, J. F., and Parker, A. M. (1994). Risk communication: Absolute versus relative expressions of low-probability risks. *Organizational Behavior and Human Decision Processes, 60,* 387–408.

Sunstein, C. R. (2002). *Risk and reason: Safety, law, and the environment.* New York: Cambridge University Press.

Sunstein, C. R. (2003). Beyond the Precautionary Principle. *University of Pennsylvania Law Review, 151,* 1003–1058.

Sunstein, C. R. and Thaler, R. H. (2003). Libertarian paternalism. *American Economic Review, 93,* 175–180.

Szrek, H. (2005). *The value of choice in insurance purchasing.* Doctoral Dissertation, Wharton School, University of Pennsylvania.

Tabarrok, A. T. (2000). Assessing the FDA via the anomaly of off-label drug prescribing. *Independent Review, 5,* 25–53.

Temple, R. and Ellenberg, S. S. (2000). Placebo-controlled trials and active-control trials in the evaluation of new treatments. Part I: Ethical and scientific issues. *Annals of Internal Medicine, 133,* 455–463.

Tetlock, P. E., Lerner, J. and Peterson, R. (1996). Revising the value pluralism model: Incorporating social content and context postulates. In C. Seligman, J. Olson, and M. Zanna (Eds.), *the psychology of values: The Ontario symposium, Volume 8.* Hillsdale, NJ: Erlbaum.

Torrance, G. W., Drummond, M. F., and Walker, V. (2003). Switching therapy in health economics trials: Confronting the confusion. *Medical Decision Making, 23,* 335–340.

Trials of War Criminals before the Nuremberg Military Tribunals under Control Council Law No. 10, Vol. 2, pp. 181–182.. Washington, D.C.: U.S. Government Printing Office, 1949.

Tversky, A., Sattath, S., and Slovic, P. (1988). Contingent weighting in judgment and choice. *Psychological Review, 95*, 371–384.

Tyler, T. R. (1994). Psychological models of the justice motive: Antecedents of distributive and procedural justice *Journal of Personality and Social Psychology, 67*, 850–863.

Tyran, J.–R. (2002). Voting when money and morals conflict: An experimental test of expressive voting. Working paper 2002-07, University of St. Gallen. http://papers.ssrn.com

Ubel, P. A. (2000). *Pricing life: Why it's time for health care rationing.* Cambridge, MA: MIT Press.

Ubel, P. A., Arnold, R. M., and Caplan, A. L. (1993). Rationing failure: The ethical lessons of the retransplantation of scarce vital organs. *Journal of the American Medical Association, 270*, 2469–2474.

Ubel, P. A., Baron, J., and Asch, D. A. (1999). Social acceptability, personal responsibility, and prognosis in public judgments about transplant allocation. *Bioethics, 13*, 57–68.

Ubel, P. A., Baron, J., and Asch, D. A. (2001). Preference for equity as a framing effect. *Medical Decision Making, 21*, 180–189.

Ubel, P. A., De Kay, M. L., Baron, J., and Asch, D. A. (1996a). Cost effectiveness analysis in a setting of budget constraints: Is it equitable? *New England Journal of Medicine, 334*, 1174–1177.

Ubel, P. A., De Kay, M. L., Baron, J., and Asch, D. A. (1996b). Public preferences for efficiency and racial equity in kidney transplant allocation decisions. *Transplantation Proceedings, 28*, 2997–3002.

Ubel, P. A. and Loewenstein, G. (1995). The efficiency and equity of retransplantation: an experimental study of public attitudes. *Health Policy, 34*, 145–151.

Ubel, P. A. and Loewenstein, G. (1996a). Public perceptions of the importance of prognosis in allocating transplantable livers to children. *Medical Decision Making, 16*, 234–241.

Ubel, P. A. and Loewenstein, G. (1996b). Distributing scarce livers: the moral reasoning of the general public. *Social Science and Medicine, 42*, 1049–1055.

Ubel, P. A., Loewenstein, G., and Jepson, C. (2003). Whose quality of life?

A commentary exploring discrepancies between health state evaluations of patients and the general public. *Quality of Life Research, 12,* 599–607.

Ubel, P. A., Loewenstein, G., Scanlon, D., and Kamlet, M. (1996). Individual utilities are inconsistent with rationing choices: A partial explanation of why Oregon's cost-effectiveness list failed. *Medical Decision Making, 16,* 108–116.

Ubel, P. A., Richardson, J., and Pinto Prades, J.-L. (1999). Life-saving treatments and disabilities: Are all QALYs created equal? *International Journal of Technology Assessment in Uncertainty, 7,* 71–87.

U.S. Department of Health and Human Services. (1996). Food and Drug Administration. Protection of human subjects; Informed consent and waiver of informed consent requirements in certain emergency research; Final rules. Title 21, Code of Federal Regulation, Part 50.24. Fed Reg. 1996; 61:51528–33.

U.S. Department of Health and Human Services. (2002). Food and Drug Administration. Protection of human subjects. Title 21, Code of Federal Regulation, Part 46.408.

U.S. Food and Drug Administration. Department of Health and Human Services. Placebo-controlled and active controlled drug study designs. May 1989.

U.S. Government (1997). Code of Federal Regulations, Title 45, Part 46 (45cfr46), revised 1997. Washington, DC: U.S. Government Printing Office.

Varmus, H., Klausner, R., Zerhouni, E., Acharya, T., Daar, A. S., and Singer, P. A. (2003). Grand challenges in global health. *Science, 302,* 398–399.

Varmus, H. and Satcher, D. (1997) Ethical complexities of conducting research in developing countries. *New England Journal of Medicine, 337,* 1003–1005.

Vaupel, J. W., Carey, J. R., and Christensen, K. (2003). It's never too late. *Science, 301,* 1679–1681.

von Neumann, J. and Morgenstern, O. (1947). *Theory of games and economic behavior* (2nd ed.). Princeton: Princeton University Press.

von Winterfeldt, D. and Edwards, W. (1986). *Decision analysis and behavioral research.* New York: Cambridge University Press.

Wakker, P. P. (1989). *Additive representation of preferences: A new foundation of decision analysis.* Dordrecht: Kluwer.

Wertheimer, M. (1959). *Productive thinking* (rev. ed.). New York: Harper and Row (Original work published 1945)

Wiener, J. B. (2001). Precaution in a multi-risk world. In D. J. Paustenbach (ed.), *Human and ecological risk assessment: Theory and practice,* pp. 1509-1532. New York: Wiley.

Wikler, D. (1994). Bioethics in health policy: What methodology? In *Principles of Medical Biology, Vol. 1A. Bioethics,* 23–36. JAI Press.

Winkelmayer, W. C., Weinstein, M. C., Mittleman, M. A., Glynn, R. J., Pliskin, J. S. (2002). Health economic evaluations: the special case of end-stage renal disease treatment. *Medical Decision Making, 22,* 417–430.

World Medical Organization. (1996). Declaration of Helsinki (1964). *British Medical Journal, 313,* 1448–1449.

Index